Carbapenemases:
A Threat to the Globe

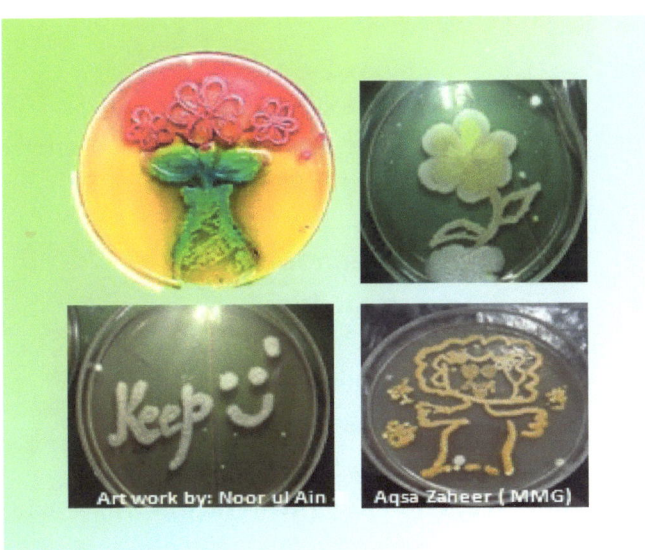

Saba Riaz, Noor Ul Ain, Farhan Rasheed,
Shahida Hussain, Muhammad Hayat Haider and
Samyyia Abrar

Carbapenemases: A Threat to the Globe

Saba Riaz
Assistant Professor
Department of Microbiology and Molecular Genetics,
University of the Punjab, Lahore, Pakistan
Citi Lab and Research Center, Faisal Town Lahore, Pakistan

Noor Ul Ain
Ph. D Scholar
Department of Microbiology and Molecular Genetics,
University of the Punjab,
Lahore, Pakistan

Dr. Farhan Rasheed
Assistant Professor
Department of Pathology, Allama Iqbal Medical College,
Lahore.

Shahida Hussain
Ph. D Scholar
Department of Microbiology and Molecular Genetics,
University of the Punjab,
Lahore, Pakistan

Muhammad Hayat Haider
Ph. D Scholar
Department of Microbiology and Molecular Genetics,
University of the Punjab,
Lahore, Pakistan

Samyyia Abrar
Ph. D Scholar
Department of Microbiology and Molecular Genetics,
University of the Punjab,
Lahore, Pakistan

Preface

This book is written to present a brief overview of carbapenemases. The authors have enlightened the characteristic features, Genetic determinants, various phenotypic and molecular diagnostic procedures for detection of Mettalo-β-lactamases. This book is the first effort from Pakistan which summarizes the prevalence scenario and diversity of Carbapenem variants worldwide and particularly in Pakistan. The book has mentioned the myths, pros and cons of various detection methodologies with their evolving trends according to CLSI guidelines.

All text, Figures, tables, flow-diagram and book cover etc included in this book is prepared by authors of the book.

All rights reserved:

ISBN-13:978-1981460021 ; ISBN-10:1981460020

DEDICATION

To all those who are the victims of vulnerable and life threatening bacterial infections!

CONTENTS

CHAPTER 1	Introduction to Carbapenemases	10
CHAPTER 2	Phenotypic and Molecular Detection Techniques of Carbapenemases	29
CHAPTER 3	Genetics of Antimicrobial Resistance Against Carbapenems	51
CHAPTER 4	Therapeutic Options for Metallo-Beta Lactamase Producing Gram Negative Bacilli	82
CHAPTER 5	References	97

ACKNOWLEDGMENTS

We show high gratitude towards all those who directly or indirectly participated in the accomplishment of this book.

We are specially thankful to Sadia Bukhari and Anam Iftikhar for their initial work

SUMMARY

The evolution of resistance to antimicrobial agents is constantly increasing and is greatly influenced by various intrinsic and extrinsic factors. Carbapenemases are beta-lactamase enzymes produced by bacterial species, capable of hydrolyzing a vast range of beta lactam antibiotics including penicillin, cephalosporin, monobactams and carbapenems. The genes encoding these enzymes are associated with mobile genetic elements particularly, plasmids, insertion sequences and transposons. *Pseudomonas aeroginosa*, *Escherchia coli*, *Proteus* spp, *Klebsiella pneumonia* and *Acinetobacter baumanni* are very common carbapenemase producing strains globally.

The problem of multidrug resistance and carbapenem resistance is spreading around the world at an alarming rate. Nowadays, several phenotypic and molecular tests are available, which are more rapid, highly sensitive and accessible for the isolation of carbapenem resistant bacterial strains. The development of antibiotic resistance depends upon β-lactamase activity, activation of antibiotic efflux systems, mutations in porins and transpeptidase encoding genes Carbapenemases including MBL hydrolyse all beta lactam drugs including carbapenems. This can have some serious effects such as limiting of treatment options, increase mortality rate, economic burden on hospitals and diagnostic centers. Combination therapy has proved effective against such pathogens. Moreover, development of more effective synthetic drugs is under way. Extensive work is required to reduce the deadly effects of this problem especially in developing countries.

CHAPTER 1
INTRODUCTION TO CARBAPENEMASES
Authored by: Noor ul Ain and Saba Riaz

In this chapter we will discuss:

1. Evolution of microbial resistance
2. Discovery of Carbapenems
3. Classification of Carbapenemases
4. Dissemination of carbapenemases through Horizontal Gene transfer
5. Different criteria of classification
6. Global Occurrence of Carbapenemases
7. Carbapenemases in Pakistan

INTRODUCTION TO CARBAPENEMASES

Evolution of microbial resistance

The evolution of resistance among microbial agents is constantly increasing and is greatly influenced by various factors including the hospitals, over population, sanitation and the spread of various microbial agents in the environment (Davies & Davies, 2010). In the developing countries, the situation is worsened by poverty, poor sanitation, ignorance of individuals, malnutrition and inadequate access to drugs. In addition, lack of research resources provided by the governmental organizations, the record of reliable data for drug susceptibility also influence the emergence of issues like drug resistance over the course of time (Byarugaba, 2004).

Important factor, contributing to the emergence of resistance in bacterial species is the acquisition of resistance genes by these bacteria from environmental bacterial species. The dissemination of resistance genes across species has also been seen to occur through agricultural lands where direct interaction of bacteria with live stocks transmits the genes directly from agricultural soil to pathogenic organisms (Levy & Marshall, 2004b). The emergence of extended spectrum beta lactamases (ESBLs) and Metallo-beta-lactamases (MBLs) in environment represents the alarming situation and major setback to antimicrobial therapy.

Discovery of Carbapenems

Carbapenems were first discovered from Theinamycin produced naturally by *Streptomyces cattleya*. Theinamycin was identified as an effective beta-lactamase enzyme inhibitor after calvulanic acid (Moellering, Eliopoulos, & Sentochnik, 1989). The class of antibiotics was developed after the emergence of multi-drug resistant isolates against members of cephalosporins like ceftriaxone, cefepime, cefotaxime, especially in the *Enterobacteriaceae*. The prevailing issue of the wide-scale resistance has posed various problems for medical science. Carbapenems exhibit a broad-spectrum activity against a variety of Gram negative as well as Gram positive bacteria. They are usually used as the 'last-line agents' in treatment of infections (Papp-Wallace, Endimiani, Taracila, & Bonomo, 2011). However, the recent outbreak of multidrug resistant isolates poses serious danger to these drugs, restricting the choice of drug.

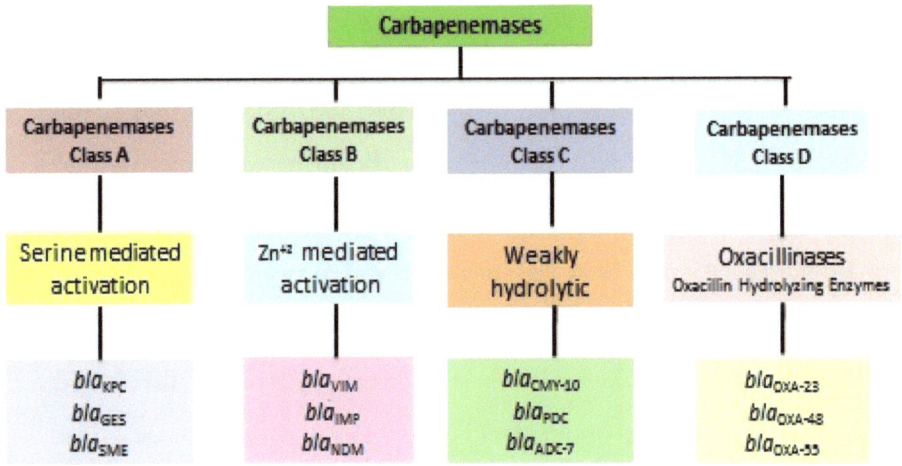

Figure 1: Classification of Crbapenamases.

Classification of Carbapenemases

Carbapenemases are the beta lactamase enzymes produced by the bacterial species, capable of hydrolyzing a vast range of beta lactam antibiotics including penicillin, cephalosporin, monobactams and carbapenems. Based on their hydrolytic activity and on molecular bases of Ambler classification, the carbapenemases belongs to class A, B and D of the β-lactamases. These potent enzymes are even able to surpass the major enzyme inhibitors like clavulanic acid, except for class A. They are inhibited by chelating agents like EDTA which is effective particularly for Metallo-β-lactamases (Thomson, 2010) (Table 1.1).

Class A Beta-lactamases

The class A Carbapenemases are serine based enzymes because according to ambler classification their hydrolytic mechanism requires active site serine at position 70. This class includes importantly, the KPC type, IMI, SME and GES enzymes (Walther-Rasmussen & Høiby, 2007). Among Class A, *Klebsiella pneumonia* carbapenemases (KPCs) were among the earliest reported enzymes. The KPCs, known to be distributed worldwide (C.-S. Lee, 2014) reported in 1996 in USA and they immediately took over other continents (Munoz-Price et al., 2013). Their production is associated with bla_{KPC} gene and these isolates are responsible for high mortality rates in clinical settings.

The *KPC* type carbapenemases are not limited *Klebsiella* spp, but there have been several reports of *KPCs* occurring in *Pseudomona*s spp. and members of *Enterobactericeae* (Bennett, Herrera, Lewis, Wickes, & Jorgensen, 2009; G. C. Lee & Burgess, 2012; Villegas et al., 2007). These *KPCs* differs from other carbapenemases in two ways; they have plasmid borne resistance mechanism and associated with specialized mobile genetic elements, the transposons. Unlike other carbapenemases, they can be transferred and hydrolyze the cefotaxime (cephalosporin) (Hirsch & Tam, 2010). Unlike others, Class A carbapenemase are inhibited by beta lactamase inhibitors like clavulanic acid and tazobactam. The detection of *KPC* is in laboratories is often complicated, because of its reduced susceptibility to carbapenem drugs ranging from slightly raised (e.g., imipenem MICs of ≤4 µg/ml) to fully resistant (Queenan & Bush, 2007).

Moreover it is usually associated with ampC β-lactamases and ESBLs, making the diagnosis crucial and critical (Munoz-Price et al., 2013). All the *KPC* enzymes, except for *KPC-2* are attributed to the gene bla_{KPC} that is conferred by the plasmid, where bla_{KPC-2} has been associated with *Pseudomonas* spp. The other *KPC* genes are rather associated with the mobile elements. The sequences similar to the sequence coding for IS1-like ATP binding proteins have been found upstream from *KPC-2* genes in *K. pneumonia* (Villegas et al., 2006) and *Salmonella enterica* (Miriagou et al., 2003). The 3'end of the tnp gene has also been found downstream to the bla$_{KPC-1}$ and bla$_{KPC-2}$ gene in *K. pneumonia* and *Salmonella enterica* (Villegas et al., 2006) whereas, no data elaborating the presence of same genetic elements in other bla$_{KPC}$ genes.

Another member of class A carbapenemases, the *SME* enzymes are named so, because of their exclusive association with *Serratia marcescens* yet, the bla$_{SME}$ are seemingly only prevalent in *Serratia* subpopulation. Also the *bla*$_{SME}$ is found to be a chromosomal gene and having a non-motile existence (Walther-Rasmussen & Høiby, 2007). The hydrolytic profile of *SME* is very closely related to *NMC-A*, however they are reported to have only 68% similarity of amino acid sequence. Till now, very little information and data has been available regarding this class of carbapenemase. The *GES* enzymes were first reported among *Klebisella pneumoniae*, the cause of infection in an infant at a hospital in French Guiana (1998) (Laurent Poirel, Le Thomas, Naas, Karim, & Nordmann, 2000).

This β-lactamase, exhibited weak hydrolytic properties against carbapenem drugs and it was named after its origin, Guiana extended spectrum (*GES-1*), followed by its variants *GES-1, -2, -4* and *-5*. The *GES-1* type, due to its low carbapenemase activity, is often considered as ESBL rather than Carbapenemase. This subtype of class A carbapenemase have been reported mainly in *Pseudomonas* *aeruginosa* (Castanheira, Mendes, Walsh, Gales, & Jones, 2004; Dubois et al., 2002; Laurent Poirel et al., 2001), yet some later studies have also reported its association with *Enterobacteriacea* (Deshpande, Jones, Fritsche, & Sader, 2006; Jeong et al., 2005). Recently the GES type enzymes have also found to be in association with *Acinetobacter baumannii* (R. A. Bonnin, V. O. Rotimi, et al., 2012).

Among all classes of carbapenemases, the first one *NmcA* was reported in member of *Enterobacteriaceae*, *Enterobacter cloacae* in 1993 in North America (Arnold et al., 2011). This sub-class was previously related to ESBLs type enzyme, owing to its properties similar to *TEM* and *SHV*. The bla_{NMC-A} is chromosomally encoded having production of enzyme at basal level with inducible expression upon encounter to the beta lactam. bla_{NMC-A} has been reported to have LysR-type regulatory regions upstream to it, similar to regulatory regions of AmpC type genes promoting the inducible expression of cephalosporinase enzyme (Naas & Nordmann, 1994).

Class B Beta-Lactamases

Molecular class B enzymes among carbapenemases are termed as metallo-β-lactamases. These are the new emerging group of carbapenemases with increasing frequency worldwide (Palzkill, 2013). These enzymes are resistant to all drugs including penicillins, cephalosporins and carbapenems but are susceptible towards monobactams (aztreonum) and EDTA (P Nordmann & Poirel, 2002). The class is named so because the enzymes in it contain zinc-metal ions in their active site. These zinc ions are essential for recruiting water molecules that are necessary for hydrolyzing target drug (Rai, Manchanda, Singh, & Kaur, 2011).

Among this class, the New Delhi metallo-β-lactamases (Yong et al.) holds immense importance. This variant of type was discovered firstly in Sweden from a patient who was in Indian descent (Yong et al.). The type of MBL was found to be closely related to VIM 1/2 type MBL sharing 32% similarity (Johnson & Woodford, 2013). Based on its geographical origin, scientists named it New Delhi metallo-β-lactamases in 2008 (Yong et al., 2009). Till now different variants of *NDM* type have been reported including *NDM-2, 3-7, NDM-2* was encountered in 2011 that differed by a single amino acid followed by other variant types (Kaase et al., 2011).

The gene responsible for *NDM-1* dissemination is *bla*$_{NDM-1}$ resides on promiscuous plasmids of 180kb and 140kb plasmids in *Klebsiella pneumonia* and *Escherichia coli*. *NDM-1* isolates are resistant to almost all types of drugs except colistin. After their discovery, *NDM-1* producing *Klebsiella pneumoniae E. coli* have been widely reported throughout the globe (Johnson & Woodford, 2013).

Another important sub-class that is of major concern is *IMP* type MBLs. This type of MBL like others is known to hydrolyze a broad range of substrates, including all extended spectrum beta lactams and carbapenems however susceptible to monobactams. The type of enzyme is not inhibited by clavulanic acid, tazobactam and sulbactam, instead it is a binuclear zinc dependent enzyme and exhibit exclusive inhibition by EDTA. *IMP* type enzymes have been divided into three major sub groups based on their amino acid similarity and difference in substrate profile. *IMP-1, IMP-3* to *IMP-7* having amino acid identity ranging from 90% to 99% are categorized as first subgroup.

The second sub group is based on *IMP-2* and *IMP-8*, having a difference of only two amino acid residues. The sub group 1 of IMP type MBLs differs from sub group 2 by 84% to 88% based on their amino acid homology. A distinctive type of *IMP*, reported from *P. aeruginosa* in Japan represents the third major sub group of bla$_{IMP}$. The *bla*$_{IMP-1}$ has been found in *Pseudomonas aeruginosa*, *Serratia marcescens*, (Kurokawa, Yagi, Shibata, Shibayama, & Arakawa, 1999; Senda et al., 1996) *Acinetobacter baumannii* (G Cornaglia et al., 1999) and members of *Enterobacteriaceae*.

The class *VIM* shares 30% similarity with IMP genes, having the same hydrolytic mechanism. Like *IMP* cluster of genes the bla$_{VIM}$ is also associated with gene cassettes residing (*aac*A4) on class 1 integron(P Nordmann & Poirel, 2002). The aacA4 codes for resistance against kanamycin, neomycin, amikacin and streptomycin (Walsh, Toleman, Poirel, & Nordmann, 2005).

The bla_{VIM} was first reported in Verona, Italy from a *Pseudomonas* pathogen in 1997 (Lauretti et al., 1999). The *VIM* variant bla_{VIM-2} was found to have 90% amino acid similarity with *VIM-1* type. This type was also found in *Pseudomonas* isolate from France (Laurent Poirel, Naas, et al., 2000). 11 different bla_{VIM} variants have been reported till now in bacterial species of different genera including *Klebsiella* (Bahar et al., 2004), *Pseudomonas* (S Pournaras et al., 2003), *Enterobacter* (Oteo et al., 2010), *A. baumannii* (R. N. Jones, Deshpande, Fritsche, & Sader, 2004).

Class D Beta-Lactamases

Class D carbapenemases comprise of oxacillin hydrolyzing enzymes termed as *OXA*. These are serine beta-lactamases by nature and are encoded by plasmid. The *OXA* enzyme family comprises of 239 enzymes among which 37 are carbapenemases while 9 are ESBLs. CHDLs (Carbapenem hydrolyzing Class D lactamases) are another name of Class D carbapenemases which show expansion in their substrate profile. These enzymes act by using efflux pumps in their membrane. First *OXA* associated carbapenemase resistance was reported in 1985 in Scotland among the clinical isolates of *A. baumanii* (Walther-Rasmussen & Høiby, 2006). OXA enzymes act against penicillins, early cephalosporins and imipenem. However, they do not hydrolyze extended spectrum cephalosporins quite easily (Walther-Rasmussen & Høiby, 2006).

Oxacillinases are categorized into extended and narrow spectrum enzymes on the basis of their resistance pattern against new beta lactam drugs (Antunes et al., 2014). The Class D carbapenemases are attributed to the genes present within the integron. These are commonly found in *Acinetobacter* and *Pseudomonas* species (Walther-Rasmussen & Høiby, 2006). According to a research, the *Acinetobacter* and other gram negative non lactose fermenter contain intrinsic genes for Class D carbapenemases which are usually OXA type. There exists a large genetic heterogeneity among different groups of OXA carbapenemases (Laurent Poirel, Naas, & Nordmann, 2010). All these *OXA* types subgroup are present in *Acinetobacter* except *OXA-48* and all are clinically very important (Antunes et al., 2014).

Dissemination of carbapenemases through Horizontal Gene transfer

The genes encoding these enzymes are associated with the mobile genetic elements particularly, the plasmids, insertion sequences and transposons. These mobile genetic elements serve as the carrier for the transmission of the resistance acquiring genes through horizontal gene transfer. Integrons are the genetic machineries capable of integrating and inserting the gene cassettes encoding resistance against multiple antibiotics. The gene cassettes are the cluster of resistance genes preceded by ribosomal binding site along with a recombination site, known as the 59-base element (59-be), present downstream of the integrated gene (Stokes & Hall, 1989). Gene cassettes for antibiotic resistance in the integrons render these bacteria resistant towards treatment by multiple classes of antibiotics, therefore eluding their use as an option for treatment.

Moreover, selective pressure of antibiotics in environment and clinical settings gave rise to large number of variants. The acquired resistance due to diverse variants of genes imparts resistance to multiple drugs at the same time. It is evident from the research conducted in the last decade that it's an endless battle to combat multi-drug resistance pathogens with the use of efficient antibiotics.

Asian countries being the epicenter for emergence of carbapenem resistance holds special concern while considering the dissemination of resistance genes. Plasmid mediated carbapenemases, being extensively versatile and associated with the bacterial mobile genetic elements, presents a high risk scenario of endemicity in the community and worldwide spread. In the past years many cases of spread have been reported, related to the importation from the foreign country.

So far plasmid borne MBLs identified includes IMP; named for being active against imipenem, VIM; Verona integron encoded MBL, SPM-1; Sao Paulo MBL, GIM-1; German imipenemase, SIM-1; Seoul imipenemase and NDM-1; New Delhi MBL enzymes (Walsh et al., 2005). Among these, IMP, VIM and NDM-1 are of great clinical interest (Bora, Sanjana, Jha, Mahaseth, & Pokharel, 2014). Both chromosomally or plasmid associated MBL genes, are known to be carried as gene cassettes incorporated within the class I integron, associated with mobile machinery of IS*CR* elements (Walsh, 2008).

In subcontinent, the origin of NDM type carbapenemases, the gene was found to be incorporated on the plasmids ranging in size between 50 to 300 Kb belonging to different incompatibility groups A/C and FIFII (Kumarasamy et al., 2010). A recent study from China (2016) has attributed the IncN plasmids to be responsible for spread of drug resistance (Du et al., 2016). The *bla*$_{OXA-48}$ is also well known to be integrated between two identical copies of *IS1999*, forming the composite transposon *Tn*1999 located on a self-conjugative mobile plasmid (Boucher et al., 2009; Carattoli, 2009; Heddini, Cars, Qiang, & Tomson, 2009). Similarly the *bla*$_{KPC}$ gene that encodes KPCs is located within the *Tn3*-type transposon, the *Tn*4401. The location of drug resistance gene on such mobile elements favors the geographic and inter-species dissemination of these genes (Arnold et al., 2011; Cuzon, Naas, & Nordmann, 2011).

IMP and *VIM*, are also important MBL gene clusters that are carried by mobile plasmid compatible to a vast array of clinically important pathogens (P Nordmann & Poirel, 2002; Walsh, 2008). The genetic analysis of IMP type MBLs have reported their existence within the specialized integrons belonging to class 1 and class 3. The bla_{IMP-1}, associated with class 3 integron was reported to be present on large plasmids. Within the Integron, this was also found associated with aac (60)-1b gene cassettes conferring resistance to aminoglycoside (Arakawa et al., 1995).

Some other studies have reported the existence of bla_{IMP-1} on Class 1 integrons, In*31* associated with *Pseudomonas aeruginosa* (Arakawa et al., 1995; Laraki et al., 1999). The In*31* belongs to group of transposons, originated from Tn402- like ancestors. It confers *aacA4, catB6, orfN and qacG*, the additional gene cassettes coding for resistance against variety of antibiotics including aminoglycosides, chloramphenicol and quaternary ammonium compounds.

The bla_{IMP-2} is known to be harbored by a different Class of Integron, having a DNA integrase gene similar to that of Class 1 and is shown to be associated with *aacA4* and *aadA1* gene cassettes (Riccio et al., 2000). So, these all specialized mobile machineries are the potential tools for dissemination and spread of resistance in the community and health care settings. The *VIM* genes are also found to be associated with the mobile elements particularly the class 1 integron, moreover a report from United states has reported bla_{VIM-7} to be carried by the conjugative plasmids of 24kb (Toleman, Rolston, Jones, & Walsh, 2004).

Different criteria of classification

MBLs are classified into different categories on the basis of different criteria. Bush classified the MBLs into Group 3 on the basis of their functional properties in 1989 (Bush, 2010). The classification was updated in 1997. Generally, MBLs can be divided into to two categories on the basis of presence of resistance gene, chromosomal MBLs and Transferrable MBLs (Walsh et al., 2005). Chromosomally encoded MBLs are those which were initially isolated from the environmental opportunistic pathogens. These MBLs can be co-regulated with some other serine beta lactamases .Whereas transferrable MBLs are spread all over the world. This is done because of the presence of special genetic machinery for transfer purposes (Walsh et al., 2005). On contrast, several MBLs are reported to be non-transferable including SPM encoded by bla_{SPM-1} related to *Salmonella enterica* serovar *typhimurium* (Toleman et al., 2002).

On the basis of sequences alignment, Class B metallo-β-lactamases can be divided into 3 further subclasses; B1, B2 and B3. These subclasses are differing from each other. Subclass B1 shows 23% similarity, 11% by subclass B2 whereas subclass B3 has only 9 conserved residues (Bebrone, 2007). Another difference in these subclasses is that subclass B1 and B3 have 2 zinc ions, present at active site whereas subclass B2 enzymes has only one zinc ion (Giuseppe Cornaglia, Giamarellou, & Rossolini, 2011). MBLs can also be divided into subgroups on the basis substrate specificity. They are group in following manner as subgroup 3a which have broad spectrum activity; subgroup 3b has ability to hydrolyze carbapenem especially and subgroup 3c poorly hydrolyze the carbapenems (Walsh et al., 2005).

Global Occurrence of Carbapenemases

Carbapenemases have widely spread throughout the globe in about 28 countries (Walsh et al., 2005). KPCs have been reported in USA, China, Italy, Poland, Greece, Israel, Brazil, Argentina, Colombia, and Taiwan (Munoz-Price et al., 2013; Yigit et al., 2001). There have been extensive outbreaks of KPCs and there is no optimal treatment available. However, the clinical data summarized by Hirsch EB *et al.*, has indicated that Tigecycline and Aminoglycosides may prove out to be effective drugs against these isolates (Hirsch & Tam, 2010).

A study conducted in India stated the prevalence rate for MBLs among clinical isolates to be 63% when these were checked against imipenem. The resistance is ever increasing and this has been demonstrated by the discovery of IMP-4 type enzymes among *Citrobacter* isolates collected in Hong Kong, China during early 2000s (Peleg, Franklin, Bell, & Spelman, 2005).

The IMP-4 type enzymes were found to be plasmid-borne and were found transferable to *E. coli* (P. M. Hawkey, Xiong, Ye, Li, & M'Zali, 2001). There have been no further reports for IMP-4 since then, when they were finally reported in 2005 in a large outbreak in Melbourne, Australia. The enzyme was found predominantly among *Serratia* and *Pseudomonas aeruginosa* isolates. These resistant organisms became the source of dissemination of resistance genes to seven other members of family *Enterobacteriaceae* and *IMP* genes became endemic in Australia (P. Hawkey, 2015).

Carbapenemases in Pakistan

The resistance pattern of metallo-beta-lactamases in Pakistan has been studied in a hospital at Rawalpindi. The study confirmed 78% isolates to be MBL producers by the use of E-strip method. Among these, *A. baumanii* were most frequent followed by *P. aeruginosa* isolates. A total of 37% of these MBL producers were detected to be susceptible to combination drug cefoperazone-sulbactam (Kaleem, Usman, Hassan, & Khan, 2010). A report from Karachi, on Carbapenem resistant *Acinetobacter* having resistance associated with class 1 integrase gene. Molecular detection techniques (sequence based multiplex PCR, Pulse Field gel Electrophoresis, Variable number of tandem repeats) have determined the presence of bla_{OXA-23} like acquired-oxicillinase gene in 50% of the isolates (Irfan et al., 2011). In Pakistan Institute of Medical Sciences (PIMS), Islamabad, PCR analysis was performed to study bla_{VIM}, bla_{IMP} and bla_{NDM-1} genes. The results revealed 23.6% isolates harboring bla_{NDM-1} gene while 25.1% and 1.5% with bla_{VIM} gene bla_{IMP} gene (Nahid, Khan, Rehman, & Zahra, 2013). From KPK, Ilyas *et al*, has reported 25.7% prevalence of MBLs in Peshawar (Ilyas, Khurram, Ahmad, & Ahmad, 2015).

Recently in 2016, Muneeza *et* al has highlighted the emergence MBLs in pediatrics patients at "The Children's Hospital and Institute of Child Health Lahore", where 59% resistance towards carbapenems has been observed and the resistant strains were confirmed to exhibit the MBLs by MHT (83.3%) (Anwar, Ejaz, Zafar, & Hamid, 2016). Similarly, a report from Faisalabad, has presented 28% resistance, towards carbapenems in *P. aeruginosa* isolates, where 87.5% were found to be MBL producer (Shan, Sajid, & Ahmad, 2015).

CHAPTER 2

PHENOTYPIC AND MOLECULAR DETECTION TECHNIQUES OF CARBAPENEMASES

Authored by: Shahida Hussain and Saba Riaz

In this Chapter we will Discuss:

1. Background
2. Phenotypic tests
3. MALDI TOF MS technology
4. Molecular Methods of Detection of CRE
5. Limitations
6. Conclusion

PHENOTYPIC AND MOLECULAR DETECTION TECHNIQUES OF CARBAPENEMASES

Background:

The occurrence of bacterial resistance, particularly mediated by genetic elements which are transferable among various bacterial isolates, most commonly *Pesudomonas aeroginosa*, *Escherchia coli*, *Proteus spp*, *Klebsilla pneumonia* and *Acinetobacter baumanni* (Sievert et al., 2013). In this regard, the clinical microbiology laboratory has to play a crucial role for the detection and separation of antibiotic resistant bacteria and exploring the mechanism responsible for the evolving the phenotypic resistance (Rhomberg & Jones, 2009). The prompt diagnostic tools are consider as utmost significance in order to select the appropriate therapeutic approach and avert the escalation of the contiguous bacterial strain in the health care setting. In this chapter, we will review the frequently used different laboratory protocols for the detection of carbapanem resistance strains of medically important bacteria around the world.

The problem of multidrug resistance in different antibiotic groups particularly, group of carbapenem is scattering around the world with an alarming rate. This potential bug affecting bacterial species of various classes and bacteria associated with nosocomial and community acquired outbreaks. Therefore, the prompt and efficient diagnosis of infected victims or colonized carriers should be considered as mandatory steps for infection control programs in order to preventing spread of this multidrug resistance bacterial group (Bartolini, Frasson, Cavallaro, Richter, & Palù, 2014). It is a complicated procedure to detect crbapenemase production due to over production of some carbapenemases isolates but susceptible, carbapnem MICs (Hsueh et al., 2010). The CLSI protocol clearly mentioned the detection methods for such resistanant strains of carbapanemase. The recognition of CP-production in any class of Enterobacteriaceae is a matter for concern for infection control team. Now a days, several diagnostic tests (approved by FDA), which are more rapid, highly sensitive and accessible for the isolation of carbapenem resistance bacteria strains. These diagnostic tests are categorized in to following groups.

1. **Molecular/nucleic acid based tests:** which are used for the detection of carbapnemase gene to study the mechanism of resistance.
2. **Phenotypic test:** most commonly used methods, to study the vitro activity of carbapenemase enzymes.

Some of the tests mentioned above are implemented directly on patient clinical specimen, but bacterial culture is a mandatory prior test in few tests.

Phenotypic tests:

In developing countries, phenotypic detection approaches or phenotypic techniques are used as a daily laboratory practice for the identification of antibiotic resistance especially isolated gram -ve nosocomial infectious agents. Here, we will cover the conventional phenotypic tests and their method of interpretation. The phenotypic tests used for the bacteria, carbapenems hydrolyzing bacteria along with other beta-lactams (carbapenemases) are under special focus of this chapter.

Imipenem (EDTA) synergy test:

Acid (EDTA) is a carboxylic acid with multiple amino acid that has ability to bind with Zinc or other metal ions and as a result inactivate the metallo-β-lactamases. Thus, this phenotypic technique is performed to isolate the CP-resistant pathogenic strains. (K. Lee, Lim, Yong, Yum, & Chong, 2003)

Boronic acid test:

This test utilizes the bronoic acids inhibitory effect or its derivatives such as 3-aminophenylboronic acid (APBA) and phenylboronic acid (PBA) for the detection of KPC production. This phenotypic test is recommended for the detection of KPC because it is easy and simple to interpret than DST.

Modified Hodge test:

In recent decades, the detection of carbapeneme resistance by using the disk diffusion approach has been gaining attention of many microbiologist or researchers. The use of three dimensional tests for detection of AmpC- class of beta lactamase was explained in the era of 1990 to 2000. The principle behind all these methods were the use of heavy bacterial colony or utilization of crude bacterial extract from isolated strains into an agar at a specific distance from the drug applied. The appearance of inhibition zone around the inoculated cup cuts was indication of presence of MBL or ESBLs. In 1976, a similar method was developed by Masuda et al., and later some alteration was made Marchiaro and Pasteran along with their coworkers. However, these methods were laborious, complicated and but easily implemented in diagnostic centers.

Among different diagnostic methods, during 1971 the test which was more common in daily practice was modified by Hodge et al., in 1978. Hodge test was published by Lee et al. This modified test was used to study the CP- production in *Acinetobacter* and *Pseudomonas species*. The replacement of Penicillin sensitive *Staph aurues* with strain of *E. coli* (ATCC 25922) and use of 10-U disk of penicillin with 10-lg imipenem disk was the major modification in pervious Hodge test. Furthermore, the addition of metals such as Zinc sulphate ($ZnSO_4$) to an Imipenem disk or into MH Agar enhanced the sensitivity of modified Hodge test was reported by Lee at al.

Although this test is simple and economical, but a high rate of false-positive results has been also detected, exclusively in Enterobacteriaceae which produce ESBLs or AmpC b-lactamases along with carbapenem-resistant due to porin insufficiency in their cell walls. The utilization of ertapenem disks and MacConkey agar showed better sensitivity for MBL producer, because of better release of β- lactamases form their cells. The addition of Zn sulphate in MH agar reduced the possibiibility of false negative results. Nevertheless , MHT till showed negative result against few NDM producers.

The major disadvantage associated with the MHT assay is prolong time; a time of 24- 48 hours are required for the appearance of first result soon after isolation of suspect-able strain of carbapenamse producing strain. Regardless of its usefulness, another disadvantage: it is only applicable for the detection of carbapnemases, in spite of unable to differentiate between different group of carbapneamse (MBL or KPC).

Although, the issue regarding the complication in the interpretation of this test gives comparatively higher rates of false negative and false positive results in some clinical isolates, the CLSI recommended this modified Hodge test as confirmatory tool for supposed carbapenemase producers. The study of literature and facts described above it has become clear that Modified Hodge test alone were not used as confirmatory test for carbapenemase production.

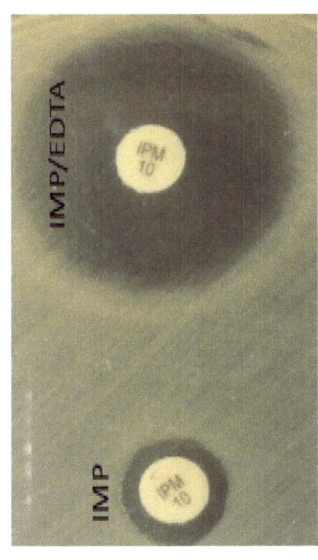

Figure 1: Double-disk Synergy test (DDST); Exhibiting the synergistic zone of inhibition surrounding IMP and EDTA disc (Noor-ul-Ain).

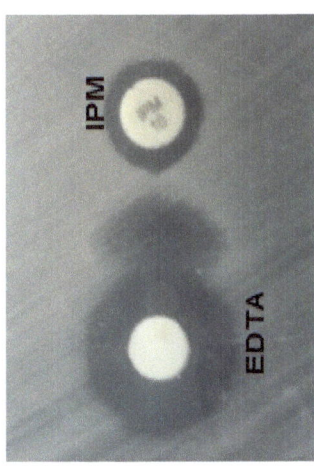

Figure 2: Combination disc test (CDST); Exhibiting the increase of >8mm in zone of inhibition surrounding IMP and EDTA disc. (Noor-ul-Ain).

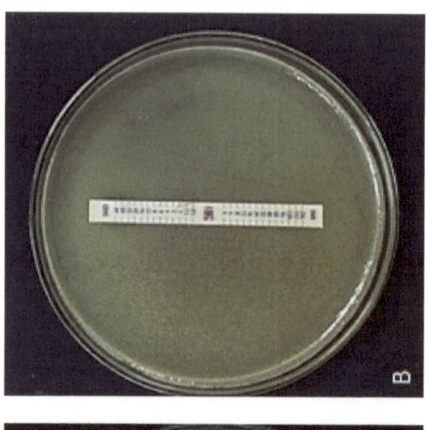

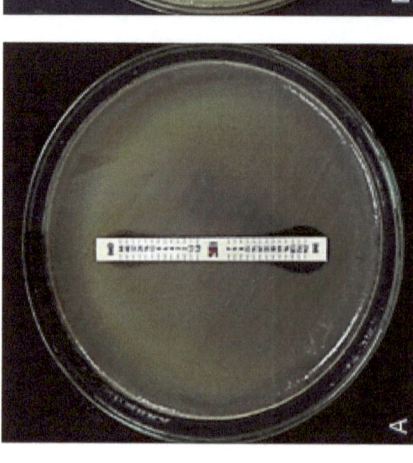

Figure 4: **MIC determination by E-strip:** (A) Positive E-Test for Demonstrating the enhanced MIC of IMP in the presence of EDTA and ratio IMI/IMD ≥ 8 for MBLs activity. (B) Not determinable Results of E-Test (Noor-ul-Ain and Samyyia Abrar).

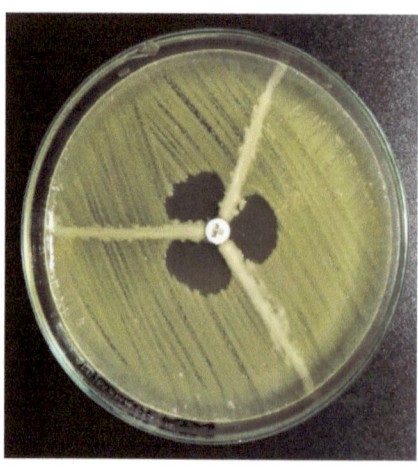

Figure 3: **Modified Hodge Test with Meropenem;** Test strains exhibiting the positive test. A clover leaf-like indentation of the control strain (ATCC25922) growing along the Test organism growth streak within the disk diffusion zone. (Noor-ul-Ain).

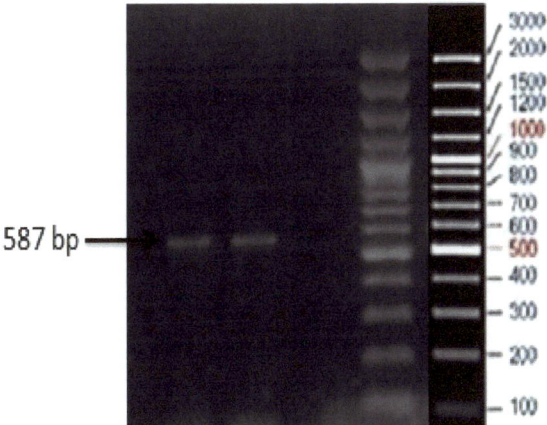

Figure 3.21: PCR Amplification of *IMP-1* Gene. Lane 1, 2 showing positive *IMP-1* with 587 bp amplicon. Lane 3 having no bands represents negative result. Lane 4 represents the 100 bp plus ladder. (Shahida Hussain, Noor-ul-Ain, Samyyia Abrar, M. Hayat Haider)

Meropenem combination disc test

In this test the EDTA and boronic acid, in a combination are applied in single culture plate. This test has been first time developed in Greece soon after the emergence of co-existence of KPC and MBL in gram negative isolates (G Meletis, Tzampaz, Protonotariou, & Sofianou, 2010). This test has ability to discriminates between different bacterial isolates associated with carbapenemas such as KPC producing, double carbapenenemase producing, MBL producing and carbapenem sensitive bacteria (Papagiannitsis et al., 2010).

In recent times, an innovative altered form of this method has been recommended for surveillance of rectal swabs cultures (S Pournaras et al., 2005; Tsakris et al., 2013). This modified method followed the same general principle. Briefly,, each swab is initially suspended in sterile saline solution, and micro-organisms are released by doing proper agitation and rotation. Subsequently, the bacterial suspension obtained is inoculated onto McConkey agar. With this test, it has been possible to make identification and differentiation of carbapenemas-producing enterobacteriacea at the time of patient admission to hospital (Spyros Pournaras et al., 2013).

Carbonyl cyanide m-chlorophenyl hydrazone (CCCP) test:

A efflux pump inhibitor (Carbonyl cyanide m chlorophenyl

hydrazine) is used to determine the CP- resistance in different clinical isolates. This inhibitor is added to MH-agar at the step of media preparation. The main principles behind this test to detect the overexpression of efflux pump which contributes to the development of carbapenem resistance (S Pournaras et al., 2005).

Detection by Use of Chromogenic Media

In this phenotypic test, two commercially available selective media such as Brilliance CRE agar and CHRO-Magar KPC (CHROMagar; BBL) are used to recognized different carbapenemase producing bacterial pathogens. Colors of the bacterial colonies are used to distinguishing the different bacterial species. The reliability of this chromogenic media has not so far been evaluated thoroughly. Nevertheless, this test can be used effectively for surveillance of various cultures in different clinical setups.

Non-nucleic acid based molecular technologies
Carbapenemase Nordmann-Poirel (Carba NP) test

Among different phenotypic detection techniques, Carba NP is more rapid and commonly used phenotypic test for the detection of carbapenamase resistance. Patrice Nordman and Laurent Poirell developed this test in 2012; primarily this test was applied on bacterial colonies. This test can perfectly isolate carbapenemase producing bacteria form carbapenemase resistance strain due to presence of non-carbapenmase mediated mechanisms of resistance.

These mechanisms involved the combined resistance mechanism (defect in the permeability of outer cellular membrane which contributed the overproduction of extended-spectrum β-lactamases or cephalosporinase) or form susceptible carbapenem strains but producing a broad spectrum beta lactamse without activity of carbapnemase (ESBLs, plasmid and chromosome-encoded cephalosporinases).

Carba NP is based on the phenomena of pH shift, using phenol red as an indicator which appeared due to presence of concomitant with IMP hydrolysis. It produces results in less than 120 minutes, while rapid yielding of positive results in some strains are also reported. Results were possible to interpreted in the time duration of <2 hours, which helps in the implementation of early containment measures. The Carba NP method has numerous benefits. It is economical, prompt, reproducible, and having high sensitivity and specificity. It excludes the necessity for performing other practices to recognize carbapenemase producing strains that are timewasting and reduced sensitivity or specificity. The implementation of the accurate test would enhanced the methodology of detection of carbapenemase colonized and infected patients. Additionally, Carba NP test has reduced laboratory workload significantly and shortened the clinical controlling of potential carbapenemases bacteria. The commercial versions of this test are R. BANERJEE AND R. HUMPHRIES RAPIDEC_ CARBA NP (BioMerieux, Marcy L'Etoile).

BOGAERTS – YUNUS- GLUPCYNSKI (BYG-CARBA) Test:

This test works on the similar principle as that of Carba NP test, but for the hydrolysis of Imipenem it uses an electro-chemical technique. This method was described by Bogaerts and his colleagues (Bogaerts, Yunus, Massart, Huang, & Glupczynski, 2016). BYG Carba is a novel and unique electrochemical test used for the prompt validation of carbapenemase resistance bacteria. Through this technique the variation in the conductivity of polyaniline which is an electro-sensing polymer layered electrode is measured. This electrode is sensitive to changing in PH and of redox reaction happening in the IMP- enzymatic hydrolysis (Bogaerts et al., 2016).

MALDI TOF MS technology is adapted in various clinical laboratories for the detection of carbapenemase resistance bacteria by detecting the carbapebemases activity. This tool relay on organism incubation in question with a CP, usually for 2–4 hrs, the quantative carbapenem detection and its degradation products. This can achieved due to hydrolysis of CP- β-lactam a ring which leads into rise in amount that can be noticeable form the innate carbapenem quantity on the MALDI TOF MS (Banerjee & Humphries, 2016).

Remarkably, prolonged incubation period are allied with false-negative outcomes, probably because of decomposing of degrading products into lighter mas, which is not detectable in queried ranges of assay. Equally, for carbapenemase with weak carbapenem hydrolytic activity, such as OXA-48, extensive incubation (> 24 hours) may be mandatory before a significant alteration in the CP-spectrum is seen (Johansson, Ekelöf, Giske, & Sundqvist, 2014; Mirande et al., 2015).

Moreover, some scholars have discovered the usage of quantitative MAL-DI-TOF to forecast carbapenem vulnerability, by associating peptide mass (a link of microbial growth), in meropenem absence or presence (Lange, Schubert, Jung, Kostrzewa, & Sparbier, 2014). There is possibility of improving results by making additional refinement in method with widespread testing protocols, but till that time, the carbapenemase detection by MALDI-TOF MS is not a sustainable choice in various medically important isolates in a laboratory. Despite the fact that, commercially at present there is no phenotypic or direct specimen test are available, some are under development, as mentioned elsewhere (Pulido, García-Quintanilla, Martín-Peña, Cisneros, & McConnell, 2013; van Belkum & Dunne, 2013).

Accelerate methods:

The direct phenotypic testing to assess the susceptibility of bacteria in the broths of positive blood cultures, **Accelerate Diagnostics,** Inc. test is utilized in clinical trials. In this method, digital microscopy of halted alive bacteria found in broths of blood cultures are utilized identify both (fluorescent in-situ-hybridization-probes) and dosusceptibility (by observing growth of bacteria or inhibition in the existence of antimicrobials). These techniques would permit rapid detection of both CP and non-CP resistant enterobacteriaceae soon after 6 hrs of a blood culture flagging positive (Banerjee & Humphries, 2016).

Molecular methods for the detection of CRE:

Surpluses of reports about molecular identification tools to detect the CP genes have been reported in the previous scientific literature published over the few past years. But only few of them are approved by FDA to use in diagnostic purpose, and the most of them are laboratory developed tests (LDT) (Table 1). The short turnaround time, specific and accurate diagnosis of CP genes, their ability to detect the resistance directly form clinical isolates without performing the culturing step makes molecular test better diagnostic tool as compared to conventional or phenotypic detection methods.

For genetic detection of CRE, the techniques based on nucleic acid-hybridization or amplification is used for the detection of genes responsible for conferring resistance. For that reason, the familiarity of definite primers (amplified nucleotides) and probes (labeled single-stranded ologonucleotides) is obligatory in demand to identify the genetic goal of concern. The nature of suspected resistance is potential factor in this technique. Polymerase chain reaction (PCR) which is very basic and simple molecular technique is performed for locating the gene associated with resistance and its expression. Genes encoding antibiotic-inactivating enzymes are one of example of PCR(Diene & Rolain, 2013).

Real-time-Reverse-Transcriptas-Polymerase chain reaction (rt RT-PCR)

rt RT-PCR is applied on those cases where resistance is directly associated with genes expression level (over and down regulation). This technique not only detects the genes presence, but also the genes mRNA expression. The end results were subsequently antagonized with expression level of control strain of same gene. With this technique, the expression of specific efflux pumps and porins can be well studied. Lastly, **sequencing** of the products of PCR are permits its conflict with the previously recognized gene sequences that are accessible in genetic databank (Fournier, Drancourt, & Raoult, 2007). Furthermore, classification, the molecular characterization or detection of mutation in a specific gene within a genetic class could be possible by this technique.

Conclusion:

The development of rapid and speedy diagnostic tools for CP has potential to enhance the bacterial surveillance, detection, and treatment therapy for CP resistance enterobacteriaceae, which is an escalating community health threat and results in restricted therapeutic choices and high mortality. Currently, many nucleic acid or non-nucleic acid based detections approaches for CRE, which are prompt and sensitive are available in market or few are under progress ofkojcxhzgj-SZi development.

However, still no molecular platform is present for detecting all possible genes conferring CP resistance. Therefore, it can be imagine by future researcher to use new testing methodologies for quick determination of CP resistance in bacterial strain of overall antibiotic resistant by mean nucleic or non-nucleic acid approaches. It helps in prompt identification of CRE and enabling clinicians to initiate effective treatment regime, hence the control infections measures and precautions can be started within hours. All above discussed points can lead to improved results, less resistance emergence, less spread of CRE and reduced health care costs.

With molecular characterization, CP genes are target treatment against specific mechanism resistance, for example the development of combination of new beta-lactam/beta-lactamases inhibitors. Although, its demand more research work on CP to demonstrate the mysterious behind the CP resistant mechanism. For optimal patient's health outcome, it should be necessary to implement rapid diagnostic methods along with anti-microbial-stewardship program involvements and other clinical decision support programs.

Pros & cons:

There are numerous pros and cons were associated in using any phenotypic or molecular detection methods for studying confrontation mechanism in Gram -ve bacteria. Phenotypic methods, demand for pure bacterial culture from a clinical specimen, therefore requiring 24-48 hour for obtaining the final report. On the other hand, molecular or genetic techniques could be performed directly from clinical samples which reducing procedure time significantly.

In phenotypic tests, the appearance of low level resistant is a problematic; therefore creating problems during the interpretation of results. In such doubtful cases, nucleic acid based molecular methods are a choice for clarifying the chances of any contribution of already accepted resistance mechanism. Besides, genetic detection technologies gives definite solution for the query of occurrence of any specific resistance contributing factor within a isolates (e.g; a specific beta-lactamase) under investigation, although with the phenotypic tests it is not possible to get only basic statistics about the involved resistance mechanisms.

Limitation:

Molecular assays however, also showed some major limitations: (1) There is possibility of screening the some known resistant mechanism more exclusively with one gene at one time approach (except utilization of multiplex PCR assay) and; (2) these methods are very expensive and their screening cost rises with increasing the quantity of resistant determinants.(X.-Z. Huang, Cash, Chahine, Nikolich, & Craft, 2012; Laurent Poirel, Walsh, Cuvillier, &

Nordmann, 2011).

The clinical and cost-effective influence of prompt diagnostics for CP-RE identification will probably depend on native prevalence of CRE and regions for upcoming research. Developments in Infectious Diseases Subsequently, the mutual and balanced practice of the accessible methods seems to be the ideal answer for the detection of resistance in clinical isolates in a microbiology lab in a cost-effective manner (Bonnin, Naas, Poirel, & Nordmann, 2012).

Method	Sample type	Gene(s) Detected	Approved by	Reference
Film-Array- Blood-Culture Identification (BioFire)	Broth of positive culture	bla_{KPC}	US. FDA CE-IVD	(Rödel et al., 2016)
Verigene (Gram- blood culture Test (Nanosphere)	Broth of positive culture	bla_{VIM} bla_{KPC} bla_{OXA-48} bla_{IMP} bla_{NDM}	US. FDA	(Ledeboer et al., 2015)
Unyvero_P55	Respiratory secretions	bla_{VIM} bla_{KPC} bla_{OXA-48} bla_{IMP} bla_{NDM}	CE-IVD	(Kunze et al., 2015)
GeneXpert (Carba-R) (Cepheid)	culture swabs	bla_{VIM} bla_{KPC} bla_{OXA-48} bla_{IMP} bla_{NDM}	US. FDA CE-IVD	(Tato et al., 2016)

Table 1: FDA-Cleared molecular tests for the detection of CP-CRE.

Table 2: Summary of Non-nucleic-acid-based- technologies for detection of CP resistance.

Method	Detection principle	Specimen type	Utilization and Use	Reference
Accelerate	Automated digital microscopy	Positive bacterial culture broth	In development	(Burnham, Frobel, Herrera, & Wickes, 2014)
Carba NP	Impipenem give color indication on hydrolysis	Pure bacterial culture	Commercial forms have obtained CE-IVD	(Österblad, Hakanen, & Jalava, 2014)
BYG Carba	Use of Electrochemical indicator for IMP hydrolysis	Pure bacterial culture	only for research purpose	(Bogaerts et al., 2016)
MALDI TOF	Mass-based recognition of products of CP degradation	Pure bacterial culture	only for research purpose	(Hrabák, Walková, Študentová, Chudáčková, & Bergerová, 2011)

CHAPTER 3

GENETICS OF ANTIMICROBIAL RESISTANCE AGAINST CARBAPENEMS

Authored by: Muhammad Hayat Haider and Samyyia Abrar

In this Chapter we will Discuss:

1. Epidemiology of Carbapenems Resistant Bacteria
2. Genetic Basis of Carbapenemase Activity
3. Genetic Expression of Efflux Pumps
4. Genetic Suppression of Penicillin Binding Proteins
5. Inter-relationship of Carbapenems Resistance Mechanisms
6. Laboratory Analysis of Carbapenems Resistant Bacteria
7. Prevention of Carbapenems Resistance
8. Current Scenario of Carbapenem Therapy

GENETICS OF ANTIMICROBIAL RESISTANCE AGAINST CARBAPENEMS

Carbapenems are β-lactam antibiotics known for their broad spectrum of activity against a large number of Gram negative and Gram positive bacteria. These antimicrobial drugs are also known as the "drugs of last resort", to be given to the patients infected with the multi-drug resistant (MDR) bacteria (Papp-Wallace et al., 2011). Carbapenems when compared to the other β-lactam antibiotics are known to be effective antimicrobial agents in-vitro against a wide range of bacteria (Raffaele Zarrilli, Giannouli, Tomasone, Triassi, & Tsakris, 2009).

Carbapenems including imipenem and doripenem are effective against Gram positive bacteria while meropenem and ertapenem are effective against Gram negative bacteria (Nix, Majumdar, & DiNubile, 2004; Queenan, Shang, Flamm, & Bush, 2010; Rodloff, Goldstein, & Torres, 2006). Multi-drug resistant *Pseudomonas aeruginosa* (MDRPA) infections are mostly treated by imipenem and meropenem, while doripenem and imipenem are given most commonly to the *Acinetobacter baumannii* infected patients (Oliver, Levin, Juan, Baquero, & Blázquez, 2004).

Carbapenems are synthetically combined with the β-lactamase inhibitors to be used as combination therapy against multi-drug resistant (MDR) bacteria (Endimiani et al., 2006; Ermertcan & Hoşgör, 2001). The combination of meropenem and clavulanic acid is used in the treatment of MDR *Mycobacterium tuberculosis* infection showing resistance towards other β-lactam antibiotics (Hugonnet, Tremblay, Boshoff, Barry, & Blanchard, 2009).

Carbapenems bind with the outer-membrane proteins (Anderson et al.) of Gram negative bacteria and enter the Periplasmic space to inactivate the penicillin binding proteins (PBPs) (Hashizume, Ishino, Nakagawa, Tamaki, & Matsuhashi, 1984; Tipper & Strominger, 1965). PBPs are the transpeptidase enzymes which perform the function of crosslinking of peptide bonds and peptidoglycan synthesis leading to the formation of bacterial cell walls (Meroueh et al., 2006). The Gram positive bacteria including *Enterococcus spp.*, *Nocardia spp.*, *Staphylococcus spp.*, *Streptococcus spp.*, and the Gram negative bacteria including *Acinetobacter spp.*, bacterial groups of *Enterobacteriaceae* family such as *Enterobacter spp.*, *Escherichia spp.*, and *Klebsiella spp.*, have developed different resistance mechanisms against clinically approved antibiotics including carbapenems.

The development of antibiotic resistance depends upon β-lactamase activity, activation of antibiotic efflux systems, mutations in porins and transpeptidase encoding genes (Limansky, Mussi, & Viale, 2002; Mena et al., 2006; Rodríguez-Martínez, Poirel, & Nordmann, 2009b). These resistance mechanisms against carbapenems differ in Gram positive and Gram negative bacteria (Papp-Wallace et al., 2011).

The point mutations or production of novel types of PBPs cause the carbapenems resistance to develop in Gram positive bacteria (Katayama, Zhang, & Chambers, 2004; Koga et al., 2009; Matsumoto et al., 2007). The development of carbapenems resistance in Gram negative bacteria in is dependent on β-lactamases, efflux pumps, loss of OMPs or porins, and mutations in genes encoding PBPs (Patrice Nordmann, Picazo, et al., 2011; Wareham & Bean, 2006). The genetic basis of these resistance mechanisms has been discussed in detail of this chapter.

Epidemiology of Carbapenems Resistant Bacteria

There are around thirty-two species of *Acinetobacter spp.*, which are responsible for multi-drug resistant (MDR) nosocomial infections (Dijkshoorn, Nemec, & Seifert, 2007; Peleg, Seifert, & Paterson, 2008). MDR strains of *Acinetobacter baumannii* have emerged in Western countries due to widespread use of antibiotics (Raffaele Zarrilli et al., 2004). The accumulation of class D β-lactamase genes in the chromosomal DNA of *A. baumannii* confers resistance to carbapenems. The carbapenems resistant strains of *A. baumannii* are emerging in Europe, North America and Latin America since last ten years. Several outbreaks of carbapenems resistant *A. baumannii* strains have been reported from France, Greece, Iran, Iraq, Israel, Middle East, Spain, Turkey, and United Arab Emirates (UAE) (D'arezzo, Capone, Petrosillo, & Visca, 2009; Feizabadi et al., 2008; Giannouli et al., 2009; Iacono et al., 2008; Marchaim et al., 2007; Meric et al., 2008; Mugnier, Poirel,

Pitout, & Nordmann, 2008; Laurent Poirel & Nordmann, 2006; S Pournaras et al., 2006; R Zarrilli et al., 2007; Raffaele Zarrilli et al., 2008).

The antibiotic resistance to carbapenems has also emerged in the *Enterobacteriaceae* family of Gram negative bacteria due to hydrolytic activity of β-lactamases. The enzymes hydrolyzing the β-lactam rings of carbapenems are known as carbapenemases (AIHidron, 2008). Most of the *Enterobacteriaceae* members belong to the normal intestinal flora of human body and their carbapenem resistant strains cause opportunistic or nosocomial infections. Mostly the *Escherichia coli* and *Klebsiella pneumoniae* since the year of 2000 are found to be associated with the worldwide spread of resistance to β-lactam drugs (Pitout & Laupland, 2008).

The carbapenems resistant *Enterobacteriaceae* (CRE) members are responsible for high morbidity and mortality in the populations of Greece and United States (Queenan & Bush, 2007). The efficacy of carbapenems is necessary to be maintained because these are the drugs of last resort. CRE have also been reported worldwide but the first CRE was reported in 1993 (Naas & Nordmann, 1994). CRE have emerged over the past fifteen years in the United States due to carbapenemase (KPC) producing strains of *K. pneumoniae* and the transposons mediated New Delhi metallo-beta-lactamase (NDM) genes transfer (Gupta, Limbago, Patel, & Kallen, 2011). The *K. pneumoniae* carbapenemases (KPCs) were first reported in 2001 from clinical samples of North California (Yigit et al., 2001).

The metallo-beta-lactamases (MBLs) including IMP and VIM confer resistance to imipenem in bacterial strains prevalent in the European and Asian populations (Sharma et al., 2016).

Oxacillinase-48 has been detected in the populations of India and Mediterranean countries (Patrice Nordmann, Naas, & Poirel, 2011). According to the findings of global surveillance programme "Study for Monitoring Antimicrobial Resistance Trends (SMART)" the NDM-1 is a major MBL detected in the carbapenems resistant bacteria isolated from Indian patients (Lascols et al., 2011). The opportunistic microorganism *P. aeruginosa* is known for its intrinsic resistance towards antimicrobial drugs and worldwide healthcare associated infections (Giamarellou & Poulakou, 2009; Livermore, 2009). The carbapenems are mostly used to treat *P. aeruginosa* associated infections, but the uptake and expression of MBL genes in *P. aeruginosa* has led to the increased resistance against carbapenems (Bonomo & Szabo, 2006; Villegas et al., 2007). The carbapenems resistant strains of *P. aeruginosa* are becoming problematic in the Europe, Mediterranean countries, Spain and China (Castanheira, Deshpande, Costello, Davies, & Jones, 2014; Gutiérrez et al., 2007; Wang et al., 2010).

Genetic Basis of Carbapenemase Activity

The antibiotic resistant bacteria produce β-lactamase enzymes as their defense mechanism which involves hydrolytic degradation of β-lactam rings of antibiotics such as carbapenems. It has been mentioned already in this book that there are four major classes of β-lactamases including class A, B, C and D. This classification is based on the biochemical structure and the catalytic properties, such as the activation and inhibition of their hydrolytic activity (Bush & Jacoby, 2010). Carbapenemases hydrolyze the β-lactam ring of carbapenems and the β-lactamases belonging to the class B are all carbapenemases. These enzymes require the activation by zinc ions (Zn^{2+}) to degrade the β-lactam antibiotics (Queenan & Bush, 2007).

Carbapenemases are wide ranging in number and have been recognized as class A carbapenemases encoded by *blaKPC* and *blaGES* genes, class B metallo-beta-lactamases encoded by *blaVIM*, *blaIMP*, *blaNDM* genes, class C carbapenemases encoded by *blaCMY-10* and *blaPDC* genes, and class D carbapenemases encoded by *blaOXA-23*, *blaOXA-48*, *blaOXA-55* and *blaOXA*-148 genes (Laurent Poirel, Pitout, & Nordmann, 2007; Walsh, 2008, 2010; Yong et al., 2009). The first *K. pneumoniae* carbapenemase as a member of class A β-lactamases was named as KPC-1 to signify its abundance in *K. pneumoniae*. Similarly KPC-2 and KPC-3 have been categorized as class A β-lactamases (Miriagou et al., 2003; Smith Moland et al., 2003; Yigit et al., 2003). *Enterobacter spp.* is an important opportunistic infectious agent and its strains have been reported to be producing plasmid encoded KPC-2 which imparts resistance against imipenem in the cases of sepsis in hospitalized patients (Hossain et al., 2004). KPC-2 differs from KPC-1 at amino acid residue glycine at position 175 than serine and KPC-3 differs from both enzymes at position 272 containing tyrosine than histidine (L Poirel & Nordmann, 2002; Smith Moland et al., 2003).

There are several carbapenemases whose crystalline structures have been studies such as class A carbapenemases including SME-1 and KPC-2 isolated from *Serratia marcescens* and *K. pneumoniae*. These enzymes are known to have specific active sites containing disulfide bonds between the cysteine residues including Cys69 and Cys238. These active sites are involved in the hydrolysis of imipenem as the disulfide bonds increase the substrate binding affinity for the enzymes (Majiduddin & Palzkill, 2005; Papp-Wallace et al., 2010; Papp-Wallace et al., 2010). The DNA sequence homology analysis of genes encoding KPC-1 and SME-1 reveals similarity index of 40% (Naas, Vandel, Sougakoff, Livermore, & Nordmann, 1994). The similarity index is 90% when the nucleotide sequences of genes encoding IMI-1 and Nmc-A produced by *Enterobacter cloacae* aligned with the gene sequence encoding SME-1 (Naas & Nordmann, 1994; Patrice Nordmann, 1998).

KPC-1 amino acids sequence alignment with other class A carbapenemases shows that there is a disulfide bond between cysteine residues Cys69 and Cys238 while the TEM and SHV produced by *E. coli* have disulfide bonds between Cys77 and Cys123 (Pollitt & Zalkin, 1983; Raquet, Lamotte-Brasseur,

Bouillenne, & Frère, 1997).

The class B β-lactamases have been further classified into subclasses including B1, B2, and B3 on the basis of their nucleotide sequence homology and three dimensional enzymatic structures (Bebrone, 2007). All these subclasses of enzymes are capable to hydrolyze the carbapenems. β-lactamases of B2 class are strict carbapenemases. β-lactamase CphA belongs to B2 subclass and activates when exposed to one zinc ion (Zn^{2+}) and becomes suppressed when exposed to another zinc ion (Zn^{2+}) (Wu, Xu, & Guo, 2010; Xu, Xie, & Guo, 2006).

The carbapenemases belonging to class C of β-lactamases are not as effective as other carbapenemases and these show very weak hydrolytic activity against carbapenems (Mammeri, Guillon, Eb, & Nordmann, 2010). The upregulation of AmpC, a class C carbapenemase is responsible for increased resistance against imipenem. The other class C carbapenems active against imipenem are very rare (Rodríguez-Martínez, Poirel, & Nordmann, 2009a; Rodríguez-Martínez et al., 2009b). The conformational changes in CMY-10 active site near amino acid residue 303 enhance the substrate (carbapenems) binding affinity which can become a significant pathway of hydrolytic degradation (Kim et al., 2006).

The mass spectrometry analysis of TEM-1 produced by *E. coli* and imipenem complex (ligand and receptor complex) also reveals that hydroxyl-ethyl moieties on C-6 of imipenem causes steric hindrance which causes functional suppression of TEM-1 (Maveyraud et al., 1998). The mass spectrometry analysis of conformational changes in three dimensional structure of enzymes and carbapenems as the substrates has revealed that class A β-lactamase BlaC and class C β-lactamases ADC-7, CMY-2 and CMY-32 remove the hydroxyl-ethyl moieties on carbon number six (C-6) of carbapenems (Drawz et al., 2009; Hugonnet et al., 2009). This removal of hydroxyl-ethyl groups causes fragmentation of carbapenem molecules which are readily hydrolyzed by carbapenemases (Endimiani et al., 2010).

Carbapenems belonging to the class D β-lactamases are oxacillinases which have been isolated from *A. baumannii* strains involved in healthcare associated infections. The gene sequence homology analysis of OXA-23 and OXA-27 reveals 99% similarity index (Afzal-Shah, Woodford, & Livermore, 2001). Similarly the gene sequence homology analysis of OXA-24 and OXA-26 shows 60% of similarity index (Bou, Oliver, & Martínez-Beltrán, 2000).

Recently the biochemical and genetic basis of carbapenemase activity of OXA-40 isolated from *A. baumannii* have been analyzed. It belongs to the OXA-24, OXA-25, and OXA-26 containing subgroup of oxacillinases suggesting a common origin. OXA-40 hydrolyzes β-lactam rings of imipenem and it is highly resistant to clavulanic acid, sulbactam, and tazobactam. These parameters of OXA-40 carbapenemase activity are associated with the presence of FGN motif instead of YGN motif of other oxacillinases at amino acid positions 144 to 146 (Héritier, Poirel, Aubert, & Nordmann, 2003). It has been tested by conjugation experiments that a plasmid (pABIR) encoded OXA-58 is responsible for emergence of imipenem resistant *A. baumannii* strains (Raffaele Zarrilli et al., 2008). Similarly the OXA-97 has been isolated form *A. baumannii* strains possessing OXA-58 like enzymatic activity but differs by a single amino acid residue (Laurent Poirel, Mansour, Bouallegue, & Nordmann, 2008).

OXA-58 isolated from *A. baumannii* is known to hydrolyze penicillins and carbapenems extensively. It contains YGN motif at amino acid positions 144 to 146. The hydrolysis of carbapenems by OXA-58 is dependent on tyrosine residue at position 144 (Laurent Poirel et al., 2005). The resistance against carbapenemases increases as a result of increased production of carbapenemase. This phenomenon has been confirmed in carbapenems resistant strains of *A. baumannii* as it possesses multiple copies of genes encoding OXA-58 (Bertini et al., 2007).

Genetics involving loss of Outer Membrane Proteins

Outer membrane proteins (Anderson et al.) also known as porins induce channels formation in lipid bilayer membranes in the form of pores through which the transport of biomolecules and hydrophilic substance takes place. Porins help bacterial cells to bind with other cells and have ability to bind with antibiotics or antimicrobial compounds. The expression of these porins varies according to the external factors such as exposure of antibiotics and drugs down-regulates the porins to escape from killing by antimicrobial drugs (Jordi Vila, Martí, & Sánchez-Céspedes, 2007). The porins have been classified in to four groups including substrate specific porins, general or non-specific porins, efflux porins and gated porins (Hancock & Brinkman, 2002; Martínez-Martínez, 2008). These porins are involved in developing resistance in bacteria and vary in their affinity for carbapenems (Riera et al., 2011). OprD porins are involved in binding and acquisition of carbapenems inside the bacterial cells through transport by pore formation in lipid bilayer membrane (Farra, Islam, Strålfors, Sörberg, & Wretlind, 2008). Mutations in OprD genes and their negative regulation are responsible for the decreased expression and affinity to bind with carbapenems (Ochs, McCusker, Bains, & Hancock, 1999; Perron et al., 2004).

Porins facilitate the transport of molecules up to or more than 1500Da and similarly the OprD porins are involved in the transport of amino acids, antibiotics, and other biomolecules by diffusion across the lipid bilayer inside the cells (Hancock & Brinkman, 2002; Tamber & Hancock, 2006). There are nineteen more porins belonging to OprD class OMPs which have been identified in *P. aeruginosa* and only the OprD facilitates the transport of carbapenems across the cellular membranes of bacterial cells (H. Huang, Siehnel, Francis, Rawling, & Hancock,

1992).

There is very little information about the biochemical properties of outer membrane proteins of *A. baumannii* because only a few OMPs have been analyzed (Martí et al., 2006). The outer cellular membranes of *A. baumannii* are less permeable than other Gram negative microorganisms due to very small number of porins or OMPs (Obara & Nakae, 1991). The cell membranes in *E. coli* are more permeable to antimicrobial drugs than *A. baumannii* due to large number and elevated expression of OMPs (Sato & Nakae, 1991). Hence the small number of OMPs and their reduced expression or downregulation is strongly thought to be associated with the development of bacterial resistance to antimicrobial drugs including carbapenems (J Vila, 1998).

The downregulation and reduction of OMPs in number is associated with the antimicrobial resistance in *A. baumannii* (Bou, Cerveró, Dominguez, Quereda, & Martínez-Beltrán, 2000; Fernández-Cuenca et al., 2003; Mussi, Limansky, & Viale, 2005). A monomeric porin HMP-AB (34636Da) consisting of 346 amino acids belongs to OMP-A family is abundantly found in *A. baumannii* (Gribun, Nitzan, Pechatnikov, Hershkovits, & Katcoff, 2003).

The nucleotide sequence homology of HMP-AB with OMP-A found in *Enterobacteriaceae* and OMP-F found in *P. aeruginosa* is mostly the same. It has ability to bind with the β-lactams and saccharide molecules of up to 800Da and transfer these substances across lipid bilayers (Nitzan, Pechatnikov, Bar-El, & Wexler, 1999). The rate of transportation is very slow but mostly the larger molecules are taken up by OMP-A and the related porins to be transported across the lipid bilayers. The molecules that are failed to be transported by OMP-F in *E. coli* are easily taken up by OMP-A porins (Nikaido, 2003).

There are other proteins in Gram negative organisms including *Enterobacteriaceae*. CarO (29 kDa) has high affinity to bind with imipenem, but mass spectrometry analysis reveals that CarO found in *A. baumannii* lacks receptors to bind with imipenem leading to the emergence of imipenem resistant strains (Siroy et al., 2005). Carbapenems resistant strains of *Salmonella typhimurium* have been observed with the downregulated or suppressed OMP-W (Hong, Patel, Tamm, & van den Berg, 2006). The information about the functioning of OMP-W in *A. baumannii*, *E. coli*, and *P. aeruginosa* is lacking and more studies are required to investigate their function and association with the antimicrobial resistance (Poole, 2002).

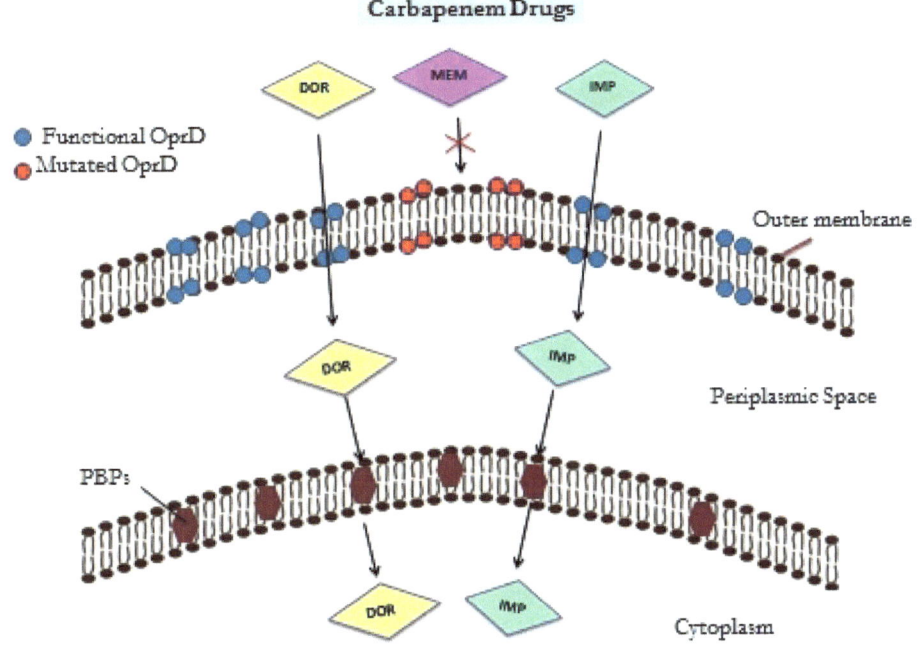

Figure: Genetic Expression of Efflux Pumps
(Muhammad Hayat Haider, Noor-ul-Ain, and Samyyia Abrar)

Genetic Expression of Efflux Pumps

Efflux systems in bacteria are multiple protein aggregates which are known as efflux transporters performing the function of transporting the toxic substances such as antimicrobial agents out of the cells. These efflux systems are found in living cells of all the organisms and their upregulation and increase in number renders bacterial cells resistant to antibiotics including carbapenems and the environmental toxicants (Papp-Wallace et al., 2011; Poole, 2002).

The antimicrobial resistance against carbapenems has been reported in *A. baumannii*, *E. coli*, and *P. aeruginosa* to be associated with the upregulation of efflux systems (Bornet et al., 2003; Giamarellou, Antoniadou, & Kanellakopoulou, 2008; Giske, Buarø, Sundsfjord, & Wretlind, 2008; Köhler, Michea-Hamzehpour, Epp, & Pechere, 1999). There are different super-families of efflux porins and systems including the ATP-binding cassette (ABC) superfamily, drug or metabolic transporter (DMT) superfamily, major facilitator superfamily (MFS), multi-drug and toxic compound extrusion (MATE) superfamily, resistance nodulation division (RND) superfamily, and the small multi-drug resistance (SMR) superfamily (Ochs et al., 1999; Poole, 2002).

The emission of carbapenems from *P. aeruginosa* is dependent on efflux pumps belonging to the RND superfamily (Papp-Wallace et al., 2011). These efflux systems consist of outer membrane porins, a cytoplasmic membrane linker protein, and a cytoplasmic membrane pump (Akama et al., 2004; Hancock & Brinkman, 2002; Misra & Bavro, 2009; Nikaido, 1996; Symmons, Bokma, Koronakis, Hughes, & Koronakis, 2009). The efflux porins OprM and OprJ in *P. aeruginosa* are attached with the cytoplasmic membranes by linker proteins including MexA, MexC, and MexX, and the cytoplasmic membrane pumps including MexB, MexD, and MexY to form a complete efflux system (Pai et al., 2001; Ziha-Zarifi, Llanes, Köhler, Pechere, & Plesiat, 1999).

There are several carbapenems which are expelled out of *P. aeruginosa* by MexAB-OprM system belonging to the RND superfamily but imipenem is not a potential target for this system (Saito, Yoneyama, & Nakae, 1999; Srikumar, Paul, & Poole, 2000; Yoneyama, Ocaktan, Tsuda, & Nakae, 1997). MexAB-OprM system is downregulated by the repressive effect of MexR repressor (Poole et al., 1996; Saito, Akama, Yoshihara, & Nakae, 2003; Ziha-Zarifi et al., 1999). There are regulatory genes including *nalC*, and *nalD* which regulate the expression of MexAB-OprM system as the mutated versions of these genes are found to be associated with the overexpression of MexAB-OprM system leading to the emergence of carbapenems resistant strains of *P. aeruginosa* (Cao, Srikumar, & Poole, 2004; Llanes et al., 2004; Lodge, Minchin, Piddock, & Busby, 1990).

The efflux of meropenem from *P. aeruginosa* is associated the upregulation of both of the efflux pumps MexAB –OprM and MexXY-OprM and their activity is associated with expression of *mexB* and *mexY* gene (Fusté et al., 2013). The overexpression of MexXY-OprM system leads to the efflux of carbapenems from Gram negative microbes (Mao, Warren, Lee, Mistry, & Lomovskaya, 2001). MexXY-OprM efflux system is not involved in mediating resistance to imipenem but possesses the efflux properties to expel the meropenem (Mine, Morita, Kataoka, Mizushima, & Tsuchiya, 1999; Sobel, McKay, & Poole, 2003; Wolter, Smith-Moland, Goering, Hanson, & Lister, 2004).

The negative regulation of MexXY is mediated by mexZ as the structural disruption due to mutations upregulate the MexXY-OprM efflux pump. Bacterial cells when exposed to antimicrobial drugs which disrupt the ribosomal function are rendered resistant to antibiotics due to upregulation of MexXY-OprM (Sobel et al., 2003; Vogne, Aires, Bailly, Hocquet, & Plésiat, 2004).

MexCD-OprJ system is another efflux system specific for the exclusion of imipenem and meropenem. The negative regulator of this efflux system id nfxB protein and the mutations in its gene are associated with the overexpression of MexCD-OprJ leading to the antimicrobial resistance against β-lactam drugs. The resistance to imipenem is highly associated with MexEF-OprN system and its expression is negatively regulated by MexT. The mutations in the *mexT* gene lead to the overexpression of MexEF-OprN. MexS is another negative regulator of MexEF-OprN efflux system (Maseda, Saito, Nakajima, & Nakae, 2000; Maseda et al., 2004).

Genetic Suppression of Penicillin Binding Proteins

All bacterial cells have a particular array of penicillin binding proteins (PBPs) which are the enzymes catalyzing the specific biochemical reactions. PBPs have been classified as high molecular mass (HMM) and low molecular mass (LMM) proteins. Both of the classes of PBPs are further subdivided into HMM and LMM subclasses A, B, and C. These proteins or enzymes catalyze the biochemical reactions of bacterial cell walls synthesis by accomplishing the transpeptidation and cross-linking of peptidoglycan chains (Born, Breukink, & Vollmer, 2006; Goffin & Ghuysen, 1998; Sauvage, Kerff, Terrak, Ayala, & Charlier, 2008).

B-lactam drugs including carbapenems specifically bind PBPs and inhibit the process of cell walls synthesis by impairing the process of transpeptidation and peptidoglycan cross-linking (Liao & Hancock, 1997). The antimicrobial resistance develops in bacteria due to mutations and reduced expression or downregulation of genes encoding PBPs. The carbapenems resistant strains of *Bacillus fragilis*, *Enterococcus faecium*, *E. coli*, *Haemophilus influenzae*, *Listeria monocytogenes*, *Proteus mirabilis*, *S. aureus*, and *S. pneumoniae* have been reported with the amino acid substitutions in PBPs encoding gens and novel PBPs genes

(Bellido, Veuthey, Blaser, Banernfeind, & Pechere, 1990; Cerquetti, Giufrè, Cardines, & Mastrantonio, 2007; Farra et al., 2008; Katayama et al., 2004; Koga et al., 2009; Matsumoto et al., 2007; Neuwirth, Siébor, Duez, Péchinot, & Kazmierczak, 1995; NOZAKI, HARADA, KITANO, & IMADA, 1984; Osaki et al., 2005; Piddock & Jin, 1995; Pierre, Boisivon, & Gutmann, 1990; Sumita & Fakasawa, 1995). PBP2 and PBP4 have been identified in *P. aeruginosa* and PBP1a, PBP1b, PBP2, PBP4, and PBP5 have been found in *E. coli* as the potential targets to be inhibited by imipenem (Hashizume et al., 1984; Song, Xie, Elf, Young, & Jensen, 1998). The morphological characters of rod-shaped bacteria are maintained by PBP2 which is a very specific target for β-lactam drugs. The dysfunction in PBP2 is found to be associated with the antimicrobial resistance in *P. aeruginosa* and other bacteria (Legaree, Daniels, Weadge, Cockburn, & Clarke, 2007).

The alterations or mutations in genes encoding PBP2 and PBP3 lead to their downregulation and impairment of cell wall synthesis. PBP3 is involved in the separation of bacterial daughter cells during the cell division. The dysfunction of PBP3 leads to the formation of filamentous forms presenting the abnormal morphology of bacterial cells. These morphological changes in *P. aeruginosa* are associated with the meropenem resistance (Blázquez et al., 2006; Giske et al., 2008; Weiss, Chen, Ghigo, Boyd, & Beckwith, 1999).

Horizontal Transfer of Carbapenems Resistance Genes

The acquired antimicrobial resistance in bacteria also depends on horizontal gene transfer also known as lateral gene transfer mediated by conjugation, transduction, and transformation involving plasmids, transposons and other mobile DNA elements (Levy & Marshall, 2004a). The transfer of genetic determinants of antimicrobial resistance within the same genus of bacteria is a common phenomenon but the inter-genus transfer of genes is also abundant among Gram positive and Gram negative bacteria (Courvalin, 1994).

Plasmids are identified by their origins of replication and antibiotic resistance genes. Bacterial cells can carry variable number of plasmids containing the particular genes representative of their total genetic makeup. Similarly the transposons also known as mobile DNAs can carry antibiotics resistance genes and can be taken up the chromosomal DNA and plasmids of the recipient cells (Alekshun & Levy, 2007). Integrons are the other genetic determinants of antimicrobial resistance which consist of multiple gene aggregates known as gene cassettes. The term super-integrons has been coined to denote the gene cassettes including about 3% of recipient cell DNA. Hence the integrons become permanently recombined within the target genomic DNAs (Mazel, 2006; Mazel, Dychinco, Webb, & Davies, 1998).

Genomic resistance islands have been defined as the sites or DNA sequences which contain the antimicrobial resistance genes. These sites containing horizontally acquired resistance genes have been identified and characterized in different strains of *A. baumannii*, *Salmonella enterica*, *Shigella flexneri*, *Staphylococcus aureus*, and *Vibrio cholerae* (Post, White, & Hall, 2010; Schmidt & Hensel, 2004). A large number of resistance islands have been identified in *A. baumannii* and one of these encodes β-lactamase OXA-23 which mediates resistance against carbapenems (Zhu et al., 2013).

The major resistance island is AbaR1 which was characterized in European Clone I belonging AYE strains of *A. baumannii*. This strain caused epidemics in France in the year 2004 (Fournier et al., 2006). AbaR1 encodes 45 antimicrobial resistance factors against different types of carbapenems. These resistance determinants include β-lactamases including OXA-10 and VEB-1 (Bonnin, Poirel, & Nordmann, 2011). The resistance island AbaR2 belonging to European Clone II contains plasmid genes encoding β-lactamase OXA-58 (Iacono et al., 2008). The resistance island AbaR3 includes plasmid genes encoding β-lactamase TEM (Adams et al., 2008).

The insertion sequences and transposons are the mobile DNA elements also known as transposable elements. The insertion sequences range in size from 0.5 kb to 2 kb and play an important role in transfer of antimicrobial resistance genes (Mahillon &

Chandler, 1998). The insertion sequences are responsible for transferring carbapenem resistance genes in *A. baumannii*. There are ISAba1, ISAba2, ISAba3, ISAba4, and IS18 which play a role in the upregulation of β-lactamases conferring resistance against carbapenems (Villalón et al., 2012). ISAba1 have been found to be associated with the transposition of β-lactamase gene bla_{OXA-23} from *Acinetobacter radioresistance* to *A. baumannii* (Laurent Poirel, Figueiredo, Cattoir, Carattoli, & Nordmann, 2008).

The spread of metallo- β-lactamase genes bla_{NDM} is also associated with the insertion sequences mediated transposition on plasmids and chromosomal DNAs of *A. baumannii, A. pitti, A. junii*, and other species (R. Bonnin et al., 2012). Generally the transposons range in size from 3 to 40 kb containing several genes. There are two types of transposons known as composite and complex transposons (Woodford & Johnson, 2004).

The molecular structure of complex transposons is different from other transposable elements including insertion sequences and composite transposons. The composite transposons are found with the insertion sequences at both ends and resistance genes in the middle. β-lactamase. NDM-1 encoding gene is found between two ISAba125 sequences forming the composite transposon Tn125. Recently a change has been observed mediated by IS26 found at both ends of bla_{NDM-1} gene in *A. baumannii* forming a composite transposon responsible for spread of carbapenems resistance (L. S. Jones et al., 2014). Tn3 is complex transposon which has been isolated form R factor (plasmid) R1. Tn2006 is associated with the carbapenems resistance by inducing β-lactamase OXA-23 in *A. baumannii* (H.-Y. Lee et al., 2012).

Integrons are the major expression systems for the antibiotic resistance genes to be recombined and upregulated in mostly the Gram negative recipient bacteria (White, McIver, & Rawlinson, 2001). The integrons as mobile genetic elements have been classified into five different groups (Gillings, 2014). Class 1 integrons associated gene cassettes containing carbapenems resistant genes have been found in a large number in *A. baumannii* strains isolated form Asian, European, and US populations (Y.-T. Lee et al., 2009). MBLs encoding genes also have been observed within the class 1 integrons such as β-lactamase IMP-1 genes (Peleg et al., 2008). Class 2 integrons have been found with the high prevalence in Argentina, Brazil, and Chile. All the transposable elements cause insertional mutations, deletions, genomic alterations, and transfer the genomic resistance islands conferring resistance to carbapenems (Mussi et al., 2005; Ravasi, Limansky, Rodriguez, Viale, & Mussi, 2011).

Inter-relationship of Carbapenems Resistance Mechanisms

The expression of β-lactamases in carbapenems resistant bacteria is not the only factor involved in the carbapenems resistance. The antimicrobial resistance arises in some cases such as

E. coli infections due to combined expression of β-lactamases with the downregulation of outer-membrane proteins (E. Lee et al., 1991; Mainardi et al., 1997; Raimondi, Traverso, & Nikaido, 1991). The imipenem resistant strains of *E. coli* have been reported with the upregulated CMY-4 and suppressed outer-membrane proteins (Bradford et al., 1997). The CMY-4 belongs to class C β-lactamases and it has been confirmed that carbapenems resistance in *E. coli* takes place due to over-expression of plasmid encoded CMY-4 and suppression of outer-membrane proteins (Stapleton, Shannon, & French, 1999).

The imipenem and meropenem resistant *E. coli* and *K. pneumoniae* strains have been reported in Turkish population with the OXA-48 carbapenemase activity and suppressed outer-membrane proteins (Gülmez et al., 2008). The resistance causing factor found in these *E. coli* and *K. pneumoniae* strains has been identified and categorized as insertion sequence IS1999 found upstream of bla_{OXA-48} involved in the upregulation of VEB-1 β-lactamase (Aubert, Naas, & Nordmann, 2003). The suppression of outer-membrane proteins OmpC in *E. coli* and OmpK35 alongwith OmpK36 in *K. pneumoniae* is found associated with the enhanced upregulation of carbapenemases (Elliott et al., 2006; Laurent Poirel, Héritier, Spicq, & Nordmann, 2004).

The inter-relationship between antimicrobial resistance mechanisms is also found among carbapenem resistant *P.*

aeruginosa. The efflux system MexAB-OprM and AmpC β-lactamase are upregulated while the activity of outer-membrane proteins OprD is suppressed in aztreonam, ertapenem, and meropenem resistant strains of *P. aeruginosa*. Imipenem and meropenem resistant strains of *P. aeruginosa* are found with the diminished OprD activity (Quale, Bratu, Gupta, & Landman, 2006).

The association between production of carbapenemases, expression of porins, and penicillin binding proteins (PBPs) has been observed to be involved in carbapenems resistance in *A. baumannii* against imipenem and meropenem. The imipenem and meropenem resistant *A. baumannii* strains are devoid of 22.5kDa outer-membrane protein (Omp7). The suppression of penicillin binding protein 2 is found to be associated with developing carbapenems resistance in *A. baumannii*. (Fernández-Cuenca et al., 2003). The absence of PB2 in *Proteus mirabilis* has been found to be associated with the less binding affinity for imipenem leading to imipenem resistance (Neuwirth et al., 1995).

Laboratory Analysis of Carbapenems Resistant Bacteria

The agar plate methods and broth dilutions containing specific concentrations of carbapenems are being used to detect carbapenems resistant bacteria (Landman, Salvani, Bratu, & Quale, 2005). The increasing prevalence of carbapenems resistant *Enterobacteriaceae* worldwide is becoming a potential threat to public health and needs proper remedy after accurate diagnosis. There are three agar plate methods being utilized for the detection of carbapenemase producing Gram negative bacteria. The first is CHROM agar-KPC, the second agar method MacI contains MacConkey's broth with 1μg/ml concentration of imipenem, and third medium MacD contains MacConkey's agar with impregnated ertapenem, imipenem, and meropenem disks. Chrom and MacI can detect specifically the resistant strains with 85% of sensitivity. MacD can be helpful in detection of resistant strains with 75% of sensitivity (Adler et al., 2011).

The antimicrobial susceptibility testing of carbapenems resistant bacteria is performed according to Clinical Laboratory Standards Institute (CLSI) guidelines by disk diffusion method using Mueller-Hinton agar plates. The phenotypic detection of extended spectrum β-lactamases (ESBLs) is accomplished by double disk synergy test (DDST), combination disk synergy test (CDST), and inhibitor potentiation disc diffusion (IPDD) method (Vaidya, 2011). The antimicrobial resistance genes are analyzed by molecular methods most importantly by polymerase chain reaction (PCR).

Genes encoding β-lactamases IMP, KPC, NDM, OXA, and VIM have been screened by PCR after DNA extraction from *A. baumannii* and *K. pneumoniae*. PCR amplicons are analyzed by gel electrophoresis and direct sequencing by kits and DNA analyzers (Del Franco et al., 2015). The transfer of antibiotic resistance genes is analyzed by conjugation experiments involving the antibiotics susceptible bacterial strains as recipient cells (Shukla, Tiwari, & Agrawal, 2004). The analysis of resistance genes also involves multi-locus sequence typing (MLST) to obtain the allele sequences by applying different methods such as Pasteur's Institute MLST scheme (Diancourt, Passet, Verhoef, Grimont, & Brisse, 2005).

Prevention of Carbapenems Resistance

There are different factors involved in the appearance of multi-drug resistant bacteria specifically the bacterial strains resistant to the antibiotics of last resort. The important factor is the disposal of hospital associated and laboratories wastes into environmental sinks and drains such as lakes and streams. These wastes should not be exposed to atmosphere and water means (Kotsanas et al., 2013). The intensive care units (ICUs) and wards should not be exposed to the clinical wastes.

The gastrointestinal specimens containing mostly the *Enterobacteriaceae* members are found to be associated with rectal swabs which should be properly disposed without contaminating the atmosphere (Chitnis et al., 2012). The proper diagnosis is recommended to minimize the development of antimicrobial resistance in pathogens by timely treatment using effective antibiotics (Anderson et al., 2007). The proper guidelines should be given to the laboratory workers to follow the pathogens control protocols and prevention practices to minimize the morbidity (Bilavsky, Schwaber, & Carmeli, 2010).

The transmission of carbapenems resistant *Enterobacteriaceae* (CRE) is necessary to be completely prevented because a very few antibiotics and antimicrobial drugs are available to treat their infections (Lowe, Katz, McGeer, Muller, & Group, 2012). The prevention can be accomplished by using physician's prescribed antibiotics with the proper dose and time through the course of treatment (Georgios Meletis, 2016). The spread of CRE also takes place by operational devices used for surgery and catheterization, therefore the aseptic techniques and newly obtained devices should be used for operations (Siegel & Rhinehart, 2007). The laboratory testing procedures should be regularly monitored by evaluation based on hand hygiene, personal safety, and waste management (Ciobotaro, Oved, Nadir, Bardenstein, & Zimhony, 2011). The reporting of new cases of carbapenems resistant bacterial infections should be accomplished by automated and computerized process so that the prevalence rates will be readily assessed. The patients of follow-up cases should not be mixed up with new cases during the epidemics (Carling, Parry, Bruno-Murtha, & Dick, 2010).

Current Scenario of Carbapenem Therapy

β-lactamases produced by Gram negative bacteria are specific against more or less all types of β-lactam drugs including carbapenems and cephalosporins. The treatment of multi-drug resistant infections can be accomplished by applying the drugs which have become last resorts including mono-therapeutics such as colistin, fosfomycin, gentamicin, and tigecycline (Miyakis, Pefanis, & Tsakris, 2011). The treatment of patients becomes problematic when treating with colistin and fosfomycin cause nephrotoxicity (Morrill, Pogue, Kaye, & LaPlante, 2015a). The tigecycline has been approved as the first line of defense against carbapenems resistant bacteria but due to its rapid diffusion from veins leads to the ineffective infection control problems (Kanj & Kanafani, 2011).

There are alternatives for the non-promising drugs such as fosfomycin and tigecycline which include oral administration of co-amoxiclav and pivmecillinam for the treatment of ESBLs positive infections (Falagas, Kastoris, Kapaskelis, & Karageorgopoulos, 2010). The patients undergoing colistin therapy are recommended to use gentamicin because studies report high resistance levels to colistin (Kanj & Kanafani, 2011). The combination therapy involving the use of another antimicrobial drug with carbapenems can be a promising treatment option. The clinical trials of treating CRE infections by combination of meropenem and moxifloxacin have given clues to use combination therapy to combat multi-drug resistance. There are several new antimicrobial agents which are in the process of clinical trials including ervacycline and alkylidenepenam sulfones which affect the activity of carbapenemases (Brunkhorst et al., 2012).

CHAPTER 4

THERAPEUTIC OPTIONS FOR METALLO BETA LACTAMASE PRODUCING GRAM NEGATIVE BACILLI

Authored by: Farhan Rasheed

In this Chapter we will discuss:

1. Beta-lactam –beta lactamase inhibitor combination
2. Polymyxins
3. Rifampicin
4. Tetracyclines and Glycylcyclines
5. Fosfomycin
    Chloramphenicol
6. Fluoroquinolones
7. Aminoglycosides
8. Newer Agents Under Development

THERAPEUTIC OPTIONS FOR METALLO BETA LACTAMASE PRODUCING GRAM NEGATIVE BACILLI

Beta Lactam antimicrobials are the most successful antimicrobial after discovery of first beta lactam drug i.e; penicillin by Alexander Fleming in 1929. Beta lactam drugs act by inhibiting the cell wall synthesis of the bacteria. They are bactericidal drug. They antimicrobial spectrum varies from simple to vide range of organisms including Gram positive and Gram negative as well as anaerobes (KONG, Schneper, & Mathee, 2010).

Beta lactam drugs consist of different groups ranging from penicillins, aminopenicillins, cephalosporins, cephamycins, monobactams, and carbapenems. Carbapenems have the most stable molecule and resist to most of the beta lactamase produced by different bacteria including extended spectrum beta lactamases. But with the emergence of carbapenemases which also includes metallo beta lactamses (Hugonnet et al.), this era of supremacy of carbapenemases has come to an end. Carbapenemases including MBL are hydrolysesall beta lactam drugs including carbapenems. Carbapenemases including MBL also make ineffective to almost all the beta-lactam –beta lactamase inhibitor combinations including co-amoxyclav, ampicillin-sulbactam, piperacillin-sulbactam, piperacillin-tazobactam, cefoperazone-sulbactam (KONG et al., 2010).

Beta-lactam –beta lactamase inhibitor combination

Because of the rising threat of antibiotic resistance, the Infectious Diseases Society of America has challenged the pharmaceutical industry to develop novel antibiotics. Specially carbapenem-resistant strains of bacteria, which are typically resistant to most or all commonly used therapeutic options and cause high morbidity and mortality (Kallen et al., 2013). As a result, the "antibiotic pipeline" has yielded an important new beta-lactam –beta lactamase inhibitor combination, Ceftazidime- Avibactam, which is gaining popularity now a days (Marshall et al., 2017). Ceftazidime-Avibactam in combination with aztreonam has very good out come against MBL producing Gram negative organisms. Both in vitro and in vivo models have yielded very good results of this combination against MBL producing Gram negative bacteria. In *vivo* efficacy of this combination was assessed in a murine neutropenic thigh infection model, which result in significant decrease in MICs when used in combination as compared to MICs of both the drugs used alone (Marshall et al., 2017). Ceftolozane-tazobactam is another beta-lactam –beta lactamase inhibitor combination active against carbapenem resistant Gram negative rods. Currently it is under phase 3 trials (C.-S. Lee, 2014).

Polymyxins

Polymyxin-Band colistins (Polymyxin-E) are sulfomethylated derivatives. They are derived from *Bacilluspolymyxa*. Colistin is a concentration-dependent bactericidal drug. The drug being a cationic peptide interacts and destabilizes the negatively charged bacterial cell membranes, leading to leakage of intra-cytoplasmic material (Taneja & Kaur, 2016). In 1950s, these drugs were first time used clinically. These drugs are nephrotoxic and also cause neurotoxicity. In the later decades, toxicity led to a substantial decline in clinical use (Koch-Weser et al., 1970). It was banned in 1970s because of toxicities (Taneja & Kaur, 2016). However with increase in prevalence of infections caused by multidrug-resistant (MDR) and extensively drug resistant (XDR) Gram-negative organisms, especially *Pseudomonas aeruginosa*, *Acinetobacter baumannii* and *Klebsiella pneumoniae* has led to a resurgence in clinical use of polymixins as a last resort antimicrobial agent.

Polymixin B and colistin are the drug of choice for the MBL producing Gram negative bugs except those organism which are intrinsically resistant to colistin like Proteus species, *Serratia* species, *Burkholderia cepacia* (Olaitan, Morand, & Rolain, 2014). But problem with colistin use is that caution is required with monotherapy. It is suggested that polymixins combination therapy should be used to increase bacterial killing and reduce the development of resistance (Bergen et al., 2015). Combination therapy of colistin with meropenem is recommended even against those organisms which are resistant to meropenem alone. It has been proven that combination therapy of colistin and meropenem have very good synergistic effects and results in significantly lowering of MICs. So combination therapy of colistin and meropenem is recommended against MBL producing Gram negative rods (Fan, Guan, Wang, & Cong, 2016).

Rifampicin

Rifampicin is believed to inhibit bacterial DNA-dependent RNA polymerase, which appears to occur as a result of drug binding in the polymerase subunit deep within the DNA/RNA channel, facilitating direct blocking of the elongating RNA (Pang et al., 2013).

Rifampicin alone itself is not used for treatment of Carbapenem resistant Gram negative rods due to rapid emergence of resistance. But in combination with colistin it is very effective and resistance development chances are also less in combination therapy (C.-S. Lee, 2014). A multicenter study was conducted in Italy as a, open-label, randomized trial comparing the efficacy of colistin and colistin plus rifampicin A total of 210 patients with life-threatening infection due to Carbapenem resistant, colistin-susceptible *A. baumannii* were enrolled. The microbiologic eradication rate was significantly higher in the combination group as compared to group given colistin alone (Durante-Mangoni et al., 2013).

Tetracyclines and Glycylcyclines

Tetracyclines are broad-spectrum antibiotics that have been available since the mid-1900s, but use in recent years has been limited by widespread resistance to these agents. Resistance generally occurs by alterations in tetracycline efflux or ribosomal protection. Tigecycline is the third generation of tetracycline, first in class of glycylcyclines, a new class of antimicrobial agents that is administrated intravenously. Tigecycline was approved by the Food and Drug Administration (FDA) on June 15, 2005. The glycylcyclines were developed to help overcome the resistance mechanisms. Because of its distinct mechanism of action It overcomes 2 types of genetic mechanisms responsible for tetracycline resistance. It is structurally related to minocycline, however, the addition of an $N,N,$-dimethylglycylamido group at the 9 position of the minocycline molecule increases the affinity of tigecycline for the ribosomal target up to 5 times when compared with minocycline or tetracycline. This allows for an expanded spectrum of activity and decreased susceptibility to the development of resistance (Frampton & Curran, 2005).

Tigecycline alone can be used against carbapenem resistant Gram negative bugs but it is a bacteriostatic drug. Different clinical trials have been conducted accessing the role of tigecycline in combination with other antimicrobials. Tigecycline-gentamicin and tigecycline-colistin combinations were proved to be more successful in clinical trials as compared to tigecycline alone. So tigecycline-gentamicin and tigecycline-colistin combinations are one of the few options available for MBL producing Gram negative bacteria (Falagas, Lourida, Poulikakos, Rafailidis, & Tansarli, 2013).

Minocycline, like tigecycline, also inhibits the 30S ribosomal subunits. It is more active against *A. baumannii* than doxycycline. Clinical data on the use of Minocycline is scarce. In a study of 8 patients treated with oral minocycline for traumatic wound infections due to MDR *A. baumannii*, resulted in clinical cure in 7 of the patients (Griffith, Yun, Horvath, & Murray, 2008). In another study, patients with ventilator-associated pneumonia due to XDR *A. baumannii* were cured with intravenous minocycline (Wood, Hanes, Boucher, Croce, & Fabian, 2003). Clinical data are lacking on the use of minocycline against MBL producing Gram negative bacteria. But it can be a good option alone as well as in combination with other antimicrobials.

Eravacycline is a new synthetic "fluorocycline" active against most Gram-negative bugs, including those with acquired tetracycline efflux pumps and ribosomal protection. It is well tolerated, with simpler pharmacokinetics than tigecycline and higher serum drug levels. Eravacycline is proved to be more potent against carbapenem resistant gram negative bacteria as compared to tigecycline. More clinical trials are need especially for eravacycline use in combination with other antimicrobials (Livermore, Mushtaq, Warner, & Woodford, 2016). **Fosfomycin**

Fosfomycin is used for the treatment of uncomplicated urinary tract infections as a single dose oral formulation. Its intravenous formulation is also used for the treatment of severe infections, like bacteremia and pneumonia, due to multidrug-resistant Gram-negative bacteria. In this form, it is usually used in combination with other antibiotics. Fosfomycin inhibits the N-acetylglucosamine-3-O-enolpyruvyl transferase, which catalyzes the conversion of UDP-N-acetylglucosamine to UDP-N-acetylmuramic acid.

This enolpyruvyltransferase is essential for any bacterium possessing muramic acid in its cell wall structure. Fosfomycin can enter the bacterial cell only by active transport. Two transport systems are known to exist, the L-- glycerophosphate system and the hexose monophosphate route. The hexose monophosphate route system is more important and has to be induced, especially by glucose-6-phosphate. Fosfomycin resistance is mainly due to chromosomal mutations. Decreased drug uptake can be caused by mutations affecting the expression of the two transporter systems. In addition, resistance can be caused by mutations in the gene coding for MurA, the target of fosfomycin. Recently, plasmid-mediated mechanisms of fosfomycin resistance have also been described, which involve the expression of enzymes capable of modifying fosfomycin by adding glutathione, L-cysteine, or H2O (Kaase, Szabados, Anders, & Gatermann, 2014).

It has been proved in different studies that Fosfomycin has very good antibacterial activity against Carbapenem resistant Gram negative bacteria. Fosfomycin in combination with colistin has proved to be a very good option against Carbapenem resistant Gram negative bacteria. In combination its efficacy is more as compared to be when used alone. An interesting finding was also noted that combination of fosfomycin and colistin was effective even against those MBL producing Gram negative rods which were resistant to fosfomycin. Also in combination therapy there are very less chances of development of resistance as both drugs have different mechanism of action. So fosfomycin alone and in combination with colistin is one the very good therapeutic option for MBL producing Gram negative rods (Albur, Noel, Bowker, & MacGowan, 2015).

Chloramphenicol

The active compound of Chloramphenicol was produced by *Streptomyces venezuelae*. It inhibits protein synthesis by binding reversibly to the 50S subunit of the bacterial ribosome. It is metabolized primarily in the liver. It requires adjustment in patients with hepatic insufficiency. Chloramphenicol has very good oral bioavailability and excellent tissue penetration. Its antibacterial spectrum is broad, including Gram positive and Gram negative bacteria, anaerobes, spirochetes, rickettsiae, chlamydiae, and mycoplasma. In 1949 after its release for clinical use, it encountered serious side effects like bone marrow suppression that restricted its use as last resort therapy. However, as it is readily available and inexpensive, it is still used in many situation as a last resort (Cassir, Rolain, & Brouqui, 2014).

Chloramphenicol is a very good option against MBL producing gram negative rods and MDR isolates. Keeping in view of comorbid condition and monitoring of Liver functions and haemtological parameters it can be used as one of the options against MBL producing Gram negative bacilli (Sood, 2016). Very limited data is available for Chloramphenicol use in combination with other drugs against Carbapenem resistant and MBL producing gram negative rod. But whenever it is used in combination it has been proved to be very effective against resistant bacteria (Arjun et al., 2017).

Fluoroquinolones

The quinolones are a group of synthetic broad spectrum antimicrobials. First and second generation fluoroquinolones selectively inhibit the topoisomerase II and lead to nucleic acid synthesis inhibition. Third and fourth generation fluoroquinolones are more selective for the topoisomerase IV ligase domain, and thus have enhanced gram-positive coverage. In early 1960 after discovery of Quinolones, considerable scientific and clinical interest was being shown for this group of antimicrobial. It potentially offers many of the attributes of an ideal antibiotic, combining high potency, a broad spectrum of activity, good bioavailability, oral and intravenous formulations, high serum levels, a large volume of distribution indicating concentration in tissues and a potentially low incidence of side-effect.

Nalidixic acid was the first quinolone to be developed but a decade later additional compounds like flumequin, norfloxacin and enoxacin became available for clinical use. Initially they were used for the treatment of urinary tract infections. In the late 1980s more active and efficient drugs, like ciprofloxacin and ofloxacin, were marketed. In late 1990s levofloxacin was started to be use in clinical practice with enhanced antibacterial activity and bioavailability. Moxifloxacin, and gemifloxacin were made available for clinical use in early 2000s with extended antibacterial and anti-mycobacterial spectrum (Andersson & MacGowan, 2003).

Fluoroquinolones are a good therapeutic option for the MDR bugs especially carbapenem resistant and MBL producing Gram negative rods. Especially fourth generation fluoroquinolones have very good antibacterial activity against these super bugs. Fluoroquinolones are very effective when used in combination with other antibacterials. They are very effective in combination with Carbapenems even against Carbapenem resistant Gram negative bacilli. They are very also very effective when used in combination with aminoglycosides. Clinical data is scarce for using combinations of quinolones with other antibacterials against MBL producing Gram negative bacilli (Tamma, Cosgrove, & Maragakis, 2012).

Aminoglycosides

Aminoglycosides are exceedingly strong, wide range anti-infection agents with numerous attractive properties for the treatment of life-threating conditions. Their history starts in 1944 with streptomycin and was from there on set apart by the progressive presentation of a progression of development of new drugs like kanamycin, gentamicin, and tobramycin, which authoritatively settled the helpfulness of this class of anti-infection agents for the treatment of gram-negative bacillary diseases. In the 1970s, the semisynthetic aminoglycosides dibekacin, amikacin, and netilmicin showed very good antibacterial activity against strains that had created resistance towards earlier aminoglycosides and additionally showing unmistakable toxicological profiles.

Aminoglycosides act primarily by impairing bacterial protein synthesis through binding to prokaryotic ribosomes. Aminoglycosides bind to the 30S subunit of ribosomes, through an energy-dependent process. This binding does not prevent formation of the initiation complex of peptide synthesis, it perturbs the elongation of the nascent chain by impairing the proofreading process controlling translational accuracy (Mingeot-Leclercq, Glupczynski, & Tulkens, 1999). Taking in view of side effects, nephrotoxicity and ototoxicity are the main drawbacks clinically for the aminoglycosides. There has been an evolution in dosing strategies largely aimed at reducing toxicity (Begg, Barclay,

& Kirkpatrick, 2001). Therapeutic drug monitoring has been used extensively to assist dosing.

Gentamicin and amikacin are the 2 most commonly used aminoglycosides. It has been shown in different studies that these two have very good antibacterial activity against Carbapenem resistant Gram negative bacteria. Aminoglycosides may be the most appropriate choice for UTIs, caused by Carbapenem resistant Enterobacteriaceae. Monotherapy of aminoglycosides is proved to be less effective as compared to be when used in combination with different antimicrobials (Morrill, Pogue, Kaye, & LaPlante, 2015b). A larger multi-center cohort study showed that aminoglycosides used in combination with meropenem, colistin, Tigecycline had significantly reduced the mortality rate among patients having septicemia with Carbapenem resistant gram negative bacilli (Tumbarello et al., 2012). When used in combination with other antibacterials, aminoglycosides can achieve synergistic killing at sub-MIC concentrations (Paul et al., 2014).

Plazomicin, a new aminoglycoside with increased resistance to some aminoglycoside-modifying enzymes, has been clinically evaluated and it may be potentially useful in the near future against MDR and XDR isolates. It is also believed that it will have improved activity against those isolates which have resistance to other drugs in this class (Paul et al., 2014).

Newer Agents Under Development

Agents under development include new β-lactamase inhibitors with activity against carbapenemases, such as MK-7655, NXL104, and 6-alkylidenepenam sulfones,[6] and several bis-indole compounds, the mode of action of which is currently unidentified. The newer flouroquinolones under development for the treatment of infections caused by MDR Gram negative bacteria include avarofloxacin and nemonoxacin. Omadacycline belongs to 9-aminomethyl class of tetracyclines, which has entered into Phase 3 clinical trials for demonstration of its broad-spectrum activity against gram-positive, gram-negative, anaerobic, and atypical pathogens causing acute bacterial skin and skin structure infections, community acquired bacterial pneumonia, and Urinary tract infections (Kanj & Kanafani, 2011).

CHAPTER 5

REFERENCES

REFERENCES

Adams, M. D., Goglin, K., Molyneaux, N., Hujer, K. M., Lavender, H., Jamison, J. J., . . . Campagnari, A. A. (2008). Comparative genome sequence analysis of multidrug-resistant Acinetobacter baumannii. *Journal of bacteriology, 190*(24), 8053-8064.

Adler, A., Navon-Venezia, S., Moran-Gilad, J., Marcos, E., Schwartz, D., & Carmeli, Y. (2011). Laboratory and clinical evaluation of screening agar plates for detection of carbapenem-resistant Enterobacteriaceae from surveillance rectal swabs. *Journal of clinical microbiology, 49*(6), 2239-2242.

Afzal-Shah, M., Woodford, N., & Livermore, D. M. (2001). Characterization of OXA-25, OXA-26, and OXA-27, molecular class D β-lactamases associated with carbapenem resistance in clinical isolates of Acinetobacter baumannii. *Antimicrobial agents and chemotherapy, 45*(2), 583-588.

AIHidron, J. (2008). NHSN annual update: antimicrobial-resistant pathogens associated with healthcare-associated infections: annual summary of data reported to the National Healthcare Safety Network at the Centers for Disease Control and Prevention, 2006–2007. *Infect Control Hosp Epidemiol, 29*, 996-1011.

Akama, H., Matsuura, T., Kashiwagi, S., Yoneyama, H., Narita, S.-i., Tsukihara, T., . . . Nakae, T. (2004). Crystal structure of the membrane fusion protein, MexA, of the multidrug transporter in Pseudomonas aeruginosa. *Journal of Biological Chemistry, 279*(25), 25939-25942.

Albur, M. S., Noel, A., Bowker, K., & MacGowan, A. (2015). The combination of colistin and fosfomycin is synergistic against NDM-1-producing Enterobacteriaceae in in vitro pharmacokinetic/pharmacodynamic model experiments. *International journal of antimicrobial agents, 46*(5), 560-567.

Alekshun, M. N., & Levy, S. B. (2007). Molecular mechanisms of antibacterial multidrug resistance. *Cell, 128*(6), 1037-1050.

Anderson, K., Lonsway, D., Rasheed, J., Biddle, J., Jensen, B., McDougal, L., . . . Limbago, B. (2007). Evaluation of methods to identify the Klebsiella pneumoniae carbapenemase in Enterobacteriaceae. *Journal of clinical microbiology, 45*(8), 2723-2725.

Andersson, M. I., & MacGowan, A. P. (2003). Development of the quinolones. *Journal of Antimicrobial Chemotherapy, 51*(suppl 1), 1-11.

Antunes, N. T., Lamoureaux, T. L., Toth, M., Stewart, N. K., Frase, H., & Vakulenko, S. B. (2014). Class D β-lactamases: are they all carbapenemases? *Antimicrobial agents and chemotherapy, 58*(4), 2119-2125.

Anwar, M., Ejaz, H., Zafar, A., & Hamid, H. (2016). Phenotypic Detection of Metallo-Beta-Lactamases in Carbapenem Resistant Acinetobacter baumannii Isolated from Pediatric Patients in Pakistan. *Journal of pathogens, 2016*.

Arakawa, Y., Murakami, M., Suzuki, K., Ito, H., Wacharotayankun, R., Ohsuka, S., . . . Ohta, M. (1995). A novel integron-like element carrying the metallo-beta-lactamase gene blaIMP. *Antimicrobial agents and chemotherapy, 39*(7), 1612-1615.

Arjun, R., Gopalakrishnan, R., Nambi, P. S., Kumar, D. S., Madhumitha, R., & Ramasubramanian, V. (2017). A study of 24 patients with colistin-resistant Gram-negative isolates in a tertiary care hospital in South India. *Indian Journal of Critical Care Medicine: Peer-reviewed, Official Publication of Indian Society of Critical Care Medicine, 21*(5), 317.

Arnold, R. S., Thom, K. A., Sharma, S., Phillips, M., Johnson, J. K., & Morgan, D. J. (2011). Emergence of Klebsiella pneumoniae carbapenemase (KPC)-producing bacteria. *Southern medical journal, 104*(1), 40.

Aubert, D., Naas, T., & Nordmann, P. (2003). IS1999 increases expression of the extended-spectrum β-lactamase VEB-1 in Pseudomonas aeruginosa. *Journal of bacteriology, 185*(17), 5314-5319.

Bahar, G., Mazzariol, A., Koncan, R., Mert, A., Fontana, R., Rossolini, G. M., & Cornaglia, G. (2004). Detection of VIM-5 metallo-β-lactamase in a Pseudomonas aeruginosa clinical isolate from Turkey. *Journal of antimicrobial chemotherapy, 54*(1), 282-283.

Banerjee, R., & Humphries, R. (2016). Clinical and laboratory considerations for the rapid detection of carbapenem-resistant Enterobacteriaceae. *Virulence*(just-accepted), 00-00.

Bartolini, A., Frasson, I., Cavallaro, A., Richter, S. N., & Palù, G.

(2014). Comparison of phenotypic methods for the detection of carbapenem non-susceptible Enterobacteriaceae. *Gut pathogens, 6*(1), 1.

Bebrone, C. (2007). Metallo-β-lactamases (classification, activity, genetic organization, structure, zinc coordination) and their superfamily. *Biochemical pharmacology, 74*(12), 1686-1701.

Begg, E. J., Barclay, M. L., & Kirkpatrick, C. M. (2001). The therapeutic monitoring of antimicrobial agents. *British journal of clinical pharmacology, 52*(S1), 35-43.

Bellido, F., Veuthey, C., Blaser, J., Banernfeind, A., & Pechere, J. (1990). Novel resistance to imipenem associated with an altered PBP-4 in a Pseudomonas aeruginosa clinical isolate. *Journal of Antimicrobial Chemotherapy, 25*(1), 57-68.

Bennett, J. W., Herrera, M. L., Lewis, J. S., Wickes, B. W., & Jorgensen, J. H. (2009). KPC-2-producing Enterobacter cloacae and Pseudomonas putida coinfection in a liver transplant recipient. *Antimicrobial agents and chemotherapy, 53*(1), 292-294.

Bergen, P. J., Bulman, Z. P., Landersdorfer, C. B., Smith, N., Lenhard, J. R., Bulitta, J. B., . . . Tsuji, B. T. (2015). Optimizing polymyxin combinations against resistant gram-negative bacteria. *Infectious diseases and therapy, 4*(4), 391-415.

Bertini, A., Poirel, L., Bernabeu, S., Fortini, D., Villa, L., Nordmann, P., & Carattoli, A. (2007). Multicopy blaOXA-58 gene as a source of high-level resistance to carbapenems in Acinetobacter baumannii. *Antimicrobial agents and chemotherapy, 51*(7), 2324-2328.

Bilavsky, E., Schwaber, M. J., & Carmeli, Y. (2010). How to stem the tide of carbapenemase-producing Enterobacteriaceae?: proactive versus reactive strategies. *Current opinion in infectious diseases, 23*(4), 327-331.

Blázquez, J., Gómez-Gómez, J. M., Oliver, A., Juan, C., Kapur, V., & Martín, S. (2006). PBP3 inhibition elicits adaptive responses in Pseudomonas aeruginosa. *Molecular microbiology, 62*(1), 84-99.

Bogaerts, P., Yunus, S., Massart, M., Huang, T.-D., & Glupczynski, Y. (2016). Evaluation of the BYG Carba test, a new electrochemical assay for rapid laboratory detection of carbapenemase-producing Enterobacteriaceae. *Journal of clinical microbiology, 54*(2), 349-358.

Bonnin, R., Poirel, L., Naas, T., Pirs, M., Seme, K., Schrenzel, J., & Nordmann, P. (2012). Dissemination of New Delhi metallo-β-lactamase-1-producing Acinetobacter baumannii in Europe. *Clinical Microbiology and Infection, 18*(9).

Bonnin, R. A., Naas, T., Poirel, L., & Nordmann, P. (2012). Phenotypic, biochemical, and molecular techniques for detection of metallo-β-lactamase NDM in Acinetobacter baumannii. *Journal of clinical microbiology, 50*(4), 1419-1421.

Bonnin, R. A., Poirel, L., & Nordmann, P. (2011). AbaR-type transposon structures in Acinetobacter baumannii. *Journal of antimicrobial chemotherapy, 67*(1), 234-236.

Bonnin, R. A., Rotimi, V. O., Al Hubail, M., Gasiorowski, E., Al Sweih, N., Nordmann, P., & Poirel, L. (2012). Wide dissemination of GES-type carbapenemases in Acinetobacter baumannii in Kuwait. *Antimicrobial agents and chemotherapy*, AAC. 01384-01312.

Bonomo, R. A., & Szabo, D. (2006). Mechanisms of multidrug resistance in Acinetobacter species and Pseudomonas aeruginosa. *Clinical Infectious Diseases, 43*(Supplement_2), S49-S56.

Bora, A., Sanjana, R., Jha, B. K., Mahaseth, S. N., & Pokharel, K. (2014). Incidence of metallo-beta-lactamase producing clinical isolates of Escherichia coli and Klebsiella pneumoniae in central Nepal. *BMC research notes, 7*(1), 1.

Born, P., Breukink, E., & Vollmer, W. (2006). In vitro synthesis of cross-linked murein and its attachment to sacculi by PBP1A from Escherichia coli. *Journal of Biological Chemistry, 281*(37), 26985-26993.

Bornet, C., Chollet, R., Malléa, M., Chevalier, J., Davin-Regli, A., Pagès, J.-M., & Bollet, C. (2003). Imipenem and expression of multidrug efflux pump in Enterobacter aerogenes. *Biochemical and biophysical research communications, 301*(4), 985-990.

Bou, G., Cerveró, G., Dominguez, M. A., Quereda, C., & Martínez-Beltrán, J. (2000). Characterization of a nosocomial outbreak caused by a multiresistant acinetobacter baumannii strain with a carbapenem-hydrolyzing enzyme: high-level carbapenem resistance inA. baumannii Is Not Due solely to the presence of β-lactamases. *Journal of Clinical Microbiology, 38*(9), 3299-3305.

Bou, G., Oliver, A., & Martínez-Beltrán, J. (2000). OXA-24, a novel class D β-lactamase with carbapenemase activity in an Acinetobacter baumanniiclinical strain. *Antimicrobial Agents and Chemotherapy, 44*(6), 1556-1561.

Boucher, H. W., Talbot, G. H., Bradley, J. S., Edwards, J. E., Gilbert, D., Rice, L. B., . . . Bartlett, J. (2009). Bad bugs, no drugs: no ESKAPE! An update from the Infectious Diseases Society of America. *Clinical Infectious Diseases, 48*(1), 1-12.

Bradford, P. A., Urban, C., Mariano, N., Projan, S. J., Rahal, J. J., & Bush, K. (1997). Imipenem resistance in Klebsiella pneumoniae is associated with the combination of ACT-1, a plasmid-mediated AmpC beta-lactamase, and the foss of an outer membrane protein. *Antimicrobial agents and chemotherapy, 41*(3), 563-569.

Brunkhorst, F. M., Oppert, M., Marx, G., Bloos, F., Ludewig, K., Putensen, C., . . . Weyland, A. (2012). Effect of empirical treatment with moxifloxacin and meropenem vs meropenem on sepsis-related organ dysfunction in patients with severe sepsis: a randomized trial. *Jama, 307*(22), 2390-2399.

Burnham, C.-A. D., Frobel, R. A., Herrera, M. L., & Wickes, B. L. (2014). Rapid ertapenem susceptibility testing and Klebsiella pneumoniae carbapenemase phenotype detection in Klebsiella pneumoniae isolates by use of automated microscopy of immobilized live bacterial cells. *Journal of clinical microbiology, 52*(3), 982-986.

Bush, K. (2010). Alarming β-lactamase-mediated resistance in multidrug-resistant Enterobacteriaceae. *Current Opinion in Microbiology, 13*(5), 558-564. doi: http://dx.doi.org/10.1016/j.mib.2010.09.006

Bush, K., & Jacoby, G. A. (2010). Updated functional classification of β-lactamases. *Antimicrobial agents and chemotherapy, 54*(3), 969-976.

Byarugaba, D. (2004). Antimicrobial resistance in developing countries and responsible risk factors. *International journal of antimicrobial agents, 24*(2), 105-110.

Cao, L., Srikumar, R., & Poole, K. (2004). MexAB-OprM hyperexpression in NalC-type multidrug-resistant Pseudomonas aeruginosa: identification and characterization of the nalC gene encoding a repressor of PA3720-PA3719. *Molecular microbiology, 53*(5), 1423-1436.

Carattoli, A. (2009). Resistance plasmid families in Enterobacteriaceae. *Antimicrobial agents and chemotherapy, 53*(6), 2227-2238.

Carling, P. C., Parry, M. F., Bruno-Murtha, L. A., & Dick, B. (2010). Improving environmental hygiene in 27 intensive care units to decrease multidrug-resistant bacterial transmission. *Critical care medicine, 38*(4), 1054-1059.

Cassir, N., Rolain, J.-M., & Brouqui, P. (2014). A new strategy to fight antimicrobial resistance: the revival of old antibiotics. *Frontiers in microbiology, 5*, 551.

Castanheira, M., Deshpande, L. M., Costello, A., Davies, T. A., & Jones, R. N. (2014). Epidemiology and carbapenem resistance mechanisms of carbapenem-non-susceptible Pseudomonas aeruginosa collected during 2009–11 in 14 European and Mediterranean countries. *Journal of Antimicrobial Chemotherapy, 69*(7), 1804-1814.

Castanheira, M., Mendes, R. E., Walsh, T. R., Gales, A. C., & Jones, R. N. (2004). Emergence of the extended-spectrum β-lactamase GES-1 in a Pseudomonas aeruginosa strain from Brazil: report from the SENTRY antimicrobial surveillance program. *Antimicrobial agents and chemotherapy, 48*(6), 2344-2345.

Cerquetti, M., Giufrè, M., Cardines, R., & Mastrantonio, P. (2007). First characterization of heterogeneous resistance to imipenem in invasive nontypeable Haemophilus influenzae isolates. *Antimicrobial agents and chemotherapy, 51*(9), 3155-3161.

Chitnis, A. S., Caruthers, P. S., Rao, A. K., Lamb, J., Lurvey, R., De Rochars, V. B., . . . Guh, A. Y. (2012). Outbreak of carbapenem-resistant Enterobacteriaceae at a long-term acute care hospital: sustained reductions in transmission through active surveillance and targeted interventions. *Infection Control & Hospital Epidemiology, 33*(10), 984-992.

Ciobotaro, P., Oved, M., Nadir, E., Bardenstein, R., & Zimhony, O. (2011). An effective intervention to limit the spread of an epidemic carbapenem-resistant Klebsiella pneumoniae strain in an acute care setting: from theory to practice. *American journal of infection control, 39*(8), 671-677.

Cornaglia, G., Giamarellou, H., & Rossolini, G. M. (2011). Metallo-β-lactamases: a last frontier for β-lactams? *The Lancet infectious diseases, 11*(5), 381-393. doi: http://dx.doi.org/10.1016/S1473-3099(11)70056-1

Cornaglia, G., Riccio, M., Mazzariol, A., Lauretti, L., Fontana, R., & Rossolini, G. (1999). Appearance of IMP-1 metallo-β-lactamase in Europe. *The Lancet, 353*(9156), 899-900.

Courvalin, P. (1994). Transfer of antibiotic resistance genes between gram-positive and gram-negative bacteria. *Antimicrobial agents and chemotherapy, 38*(7), 1447.

Cuzon, G., Naas, T., & Nordmann, P. (2011). Functional characterization of Tn4401, a Tn3-based transposon involved in blaKPC gene mobilization. *Antimicrobial agents and chemotherapy, 55*(11), 5370-5373.

D'arezzo, S., Capone, A., Petrosillo, N., & Visca, P. (2009). Epidemic multidrug-resistant Acinetobacter baumannii related to European clonal types I and II in Rome (Italy). *Clinical Microbiology and Infection, 15*(4), 347-357.

Davies, J., & Davies, D. (2010). Origins and evolution of antibiotic resistance. *Microbiology and Molecular Biology Reviews, 74*(3), 417-433.

Del Franco, M., Paone, L., Novati, R., Giacomazzi, C. G., Bagattini, M., Galotto, C., . . . Zarrilli, R. (2015). Molecular epidemiology of carbapenem resistant Enterobacteriaceae in Valle d'Aosta region, Italy, shows the emergence of KPC-2 producing Klebsiella pneumoniae clonal complex 101 (ST101 and ST1789). *BMC microbiology, 15*(1), 260.

Deshpande, L. M., Jones, R. N., Fritsche, T. R., & Sader, H. S. (2006). Occurrence and characterization of carbapenemase-producing Enterobacteriaceae: report from the SENTRY Antimicrobial Surveillance Program (2000–2004). *Microbial Drug Resistance, 12*(4), 223-230.

Diancourt, L., Passet, V., Verhoef, J., Grimont, P. A., & Brisse, S. (2005). Multilocus sequence typing of Klebsiella pneumoniae nosocomial isolates. *Journal of clinical microbiology, 43*(8), 4178-4182.

Diene, S. M., & Rolain, J.-M. (2013). Investigation of antibiotic resistance in the genomic era of multidrug-resistant Gram-negative bacilli, especially Enterobacteriaceae, Pseudomonas and Acinetobacter. *Expert review of anti-infective therapy, 11*(3), 277-296.

Dijkshoorn, L., Nemec, A., & Seifert, H. (2007). An increasing threat in hospitals: multidrug-resistant Acinetobacter baumannii. *Nature Reviews Microbiology, 5*(12), 939-951.

Drawz, S. M., Babic, M., Bethel, C. R., Taracila, M., Distler, A. M., Ori, C., . . . Bonomo, R. A. (2009). Inhibition of the class C β-lactamase from Acinetobacter spp.: insights into effective inhibitor design. *Biochemistry, 49*(2), 329-340.

Du, J., Li, B., Cao, J., Wu, Q., Chen, H., Hou, Y., . . . Zhou, T. (2016). Molecular Characterization and Epidemiologic Study of NDM-1-Producing Extensively Drug-Resistant Escherichia coli. *Microbial Drug Resistance*.

Dubois, V., Poirel, L., Marie, C., Arpin, C., Nordmann, P., & Quentin, C. (2002). Molecular characterization of a novel class 1 integron containing blaGES-1 and a fused product of aac (3)-Ib/aac (6")-Ib" gene cassettes in Pseudomonas aeruginosa. *Antimicrobial agents and chemotherapy, 46*(3), 638-645.

Durante-Mangoni, E., Signoriello, G., Andini, R., Mattei, A., De Cristoforo, M., Murino, P., . . . Galdieri, N. (2013). Colistin and rifampicin compared with colistin alone for the treatment of serious infections due to extensively drug-resistant Acinetobacter baumannii. A multicentre, randomised, clinical trial. *Clinical infectious diseases*, cit253.

Elliott, E., Brink, A. J., van Greune, J., Els, Z., Woodford, N., Turton, J., . . . Livermore, D. M. (2006). In vivo development of ertapenem resistance in a patient with pneumonia caused by Klebsiella pneumoniae with an extended-spectrum β-lactamase. *Clinical infectious diseases, 42*(11), e95-e98.

Endimiani, A., Doi, Y., Bethel, C. R., Taracila, M., Adams-Haduch, J. M., O'Keefe, A., . . . Page, M. G. (2010). Enhancing resistance to cephalosporins in class C β-lactamases: impact

of Gly214Glu in CMY-2. *Biochemistry, 49*(5), 1014-1023.
Endimiani, A., Luzzaro, F., Pini, B., Amicosante, G., Rossolini, G. M., & Toniolo, A. Q. (2006). Pseudomonas aeruginosa bloodstream infections: risk factors and treatment outcome related to expression of the PER-1 extended-spectrum beta-lactamase. *BMC infectious diseases, 6*(1), 52.
Ermertcan, Ş., & Hoşgör, M. (2001). Investigation of synergism of meropenem and ciprofloxacin against Pseudomonas aeruginosa and Acinetobacter strains isolated from intensive care unit infections. *Scandinavian journal of infectious diseases, 33*(11), 818-821.
Falagas, M. E., Kastoris, A. C., Kapaskelis, A. M., & Karageorgopoulos, D. E. (2010). Fosfomycin for the treatment of multidrug-resistant, including extended-spectrum β-lactamase producing, Enterobacteriaceae infections: a systematic review. *The Lancet infectious diseases, 10*(1), 43-50.
Falagas, M. E., Lourida, P., Poulikakos, P., Rafailidis, P. I., & Tansarli, G. S. (2013). Antibiotic treatment of infections due to carbapenem-resistant Enterobacteriaceae: systematic evaluation of the available evidence. *Antimicrobial agents and chemotherapy*, AAC. 01222-01213.
Fan, B., Guan, J., Wang, X., & Cong, Y. (2016). Activity of colistin in combination with meropenem, tigecycline, fosfomycin, fusidic acid, rifampin or sulbactam against extensively drug-resistant Acinetobacter baumannii in a murine thigh-infection model. *PLoS One, 11*(6), e0157757.
Farra, A., Islam, S., Strålfors, A., Sörberg, M., & Wretlind, B. (2008). Role of outer membrane protein OprD and penicillin-binding proteins in resistance of Pseudomonas aeruginosa to imipenem and meropenem. *International journal of antimicrobial agents, 31*(5), 427-433.
Feizabadi, M., Fathollahzadeh, B., Taherikalani, M., Rasoolinejad, M., Sadeghifard, N., Aligholi, M., . . . Mohammadi-Yegane, S. (2008). Antimicrobial susceptibility patterns and distribution of blaOXA genes among Acinetobacter spp. Isolated from patients at Tehran hospitals. *Jpn J Infect Dis, 61*(4), 274-278.
Fernández-Cuenca, F., Martínez-Martínez, L., Conejo, M. C.,

Ayala, J. A., Perea, E. J., & Pascual, A. (2003). Relationship between β-lactamase production, outer membrane protein and penicillin-binding protein profiles on the activity of carbapenems against clinical isolates of Acinetobacter baumannii. *Journal of Antimicrobial Chemotherapy, 51*(3), 565-574.

Fournier, P.-E., Drancourt, M., & Raoult, D. (2007). Bacterial genome sequencing and its use in infectious diseases. *The Lancet infectious diseases, 7*(11), 711-723.

Fournier, P.-E., Vallenet, D., Barbe, V., Audic, S., Ogata, H., Poirel, L., . . . Abergel, C. (2006). Comparative genomics of multidrug resistance in Acinetobacter baumannii. *PLoS genetics, 2*(1), e7.

Frampton, J. E., & Curran, M. P. (2005). Tigecycline. *Drugs, 65*(18), 2623-2635.

Fusté, E., López-Jiménez, L., Segura, C., Gainza, E., Vinuesa, T., & Viñas, M. (2013). Carbapenem-resistance mechanisms of multidrug-resistant Pseudomonas aeruginosa. *Journal of medical microbiology, 62*(9), 1317-1325.

Giamarellou, H., Antoniadou, A., & Kanellakopoulou, K. (2008). Acinetobacter baumannii: a universal threat to public health? *International journal of antimicrobial agents, 32*(2), 106-119.

Giamarellou, H., & Poulakou, G. (2009). Multidrug-resistant gram-negative infections. *Drugs, 69*(14), 1879-1901.

Giannouli, M., Tomasone, F., Agodi, A., Vahaboglu, H., Daoud, Z., Triassi, M., . . . Zarrilli, R. (2009). Molecular epidemiology of carbapenem-resistant Acinetobacter baumannii strains in intensive care units of multiple Mediterranean hospitals. *Journal of antimicrobial chemotherapy, 63*(4), 828-830.

Gillings, M. R. (2014). Integrons: past, present, and future. *Microbiology and Molecular Biology Reviews, 78*(2), 257-277.

Giske, C. G., Buarø, L., Sundsfjord, A., & Wretlind, B. (2008). Alterations of porin, pumps, and penicillin-binding proteins in carbapenem resistant clinical isolates of Pseudomonas aeruginosa. *Microbial Drug Resistance, 14*(1), 23-30.

Goffin, C., & Ghuysen, J.-M. (1998). Multimodular penicillin-binding proteins: an enigmatic family of orthologs and paralogs. *Microbiology and Molecular Biology Reviews, 62*(4), 1079-1093.

Gribun, A., Nitzan, Y., Pechatnikov, I., Hershkovits, G., & Katcoff, D. J. (2003). Molecular and structural characterization of the HMP-AB gene encoding a pore-forming protein from a clinical isolate of Acinetobacter baumannii. *Current microbiology, 47*(5), 434-443.

Griffith, M. E., Yun, H. C., Horvath, L. L., & Murray, C. K. (2008). Minocycline therapy for traumatic wound infections caused by the multidrug-resistant Acinetobacter baumannii-Acinetobacter calcoaceticus complex. *Infectious Diseases in Clinical Practice, 16*(1), 16-19.

Gülmez, D., Woodford, N., Palepou, M.-F. I., Mushtaq, S., Metan, G., Yakupogullari, Y., . . . Livermore, D. M. (2008). Carbapenem-resistant Escherichia coli and Klebsiella pneumoniae isolates from Turkey with OXA-48-like carbapenemases and outer membrane protein loss. *International journal of antimicrobial agents, 31*(6), 523-526.

Gupta, N., Limbago, B. M., Patel, J. B., & Kallen, A. J. (2011). Carbapenem-resistant Enterobacteriaceae: epidemiology and prevention. *Clinical infectious diseases, 53*(1), 60-67.

Gutiérrez, O., Juan, C., Cercenado, E., Navarro, F., Bouza, E., Coll, P., . . . Oliver, A. (2007). Molecular epidemiology and mechanisms of carbapenem resistance in Pseudomonas aeruginosa isolates from Spanish hospitals. *Antimicrobial agents and chemotherapy, 51*(12), 4329-4335.

Hancock, R. E., & Brinkman, F. S. (2002). Function of Pseudomonas porins in uptake and efflux. *Annual Reviews in Microbiology, 56*(1), 17-38.

HASHIZUME, T., ISHINO, F., NAKAGAWA, J.-I., TAMAKI, S., & MATSUHASHI, M. (1984). Studies on the mechanism of action of imipenem (N-formimidoylthienamycin) in vitro: binding to the penicillin-binding proteins (PBPs) in Escherichia coli and Pseudomonas aeruginosa, and inhibition of enzyme activities due to the PBPs in E. coli. *The Journal of antibiotics, 37*(4), 394-400.

Hawkey, P. (2015). Multidrug-resistant Gram-negative bacteria: a product of globalization. *Journal of Hospital Infection, 89*(4), 241-247.

Hawkey, P. M., Xiong, J., Ye, H., Li, H., & M'Zali, F. H. (2001). Occurrence of a new metallo-β-lactamase IMP-4 carried on a conjugative plasmid in Citrobacter youngae from the People's Republic of China. *FEMS microbiology letters, 194*(1), 53-57.

Heddini, A., Cars, O., Qiang, S., & Tomson, G. (2009). Antibiotic resistance in China—a major future challenge. *The Lancet, 373*(9657), 30.

Héritier, C., Poirel, L., Aubert, D., & Nordmann, P. (2003). Genetic and functional analysis of the chromosome-encoded carbapenem-hydrolyzing oxacillinase OXA-40 of Acinetobacter baumannii. *Antimicrobial agents and chemotherapy, 47*(1), 268-273.

Hirsch, E. B., & Tam, V. H. (2010). Detection and treatment options for Klebsiella pneumoniae carbapenemases (KPCs): an emerging cause of multidrug-resistant infection. *Journal of antimicrobial chemotherapy*, dkq108.

Hong, H., Patel, D. R., Tamm, L. K., & van den Berg, B. (2006). The outer membrane protein OmpW forms an eight-stranded β-barrel with a hydrophobic channel. *Journal of biological chemistry, 281*(11), 7568-7577.

Hossain, A., Ferraro, M., Pino, R. M., Dew, R., Moland, E., Lockhart, T., . . . Hanson, N. (2004). Plasmid-mediated carbapenem-hydrolyzing enzyme KPC-2 in an Enterobacter sp. *Antimicrobial agents and chemotherapy, 48*(11), 4438-4440.

Hrabák, J., Walková, R., Študentová, V., Chudáčková, E., & Bergerová, T. (2011). Carbapenemase activity detection by matrix-assisted laser desorption ionization-time of flight mass spectrometry. *Journal of clinical microbiology, 49*(9), 3222-3227.

Hsueh, P.-R., Ko, W.-C., Wu, J.-J., Lu, J.-J., Wang, F.-D., Wu, H.-Y., . . . Teng, L.-J. (2010). Consensus statement on the adherence to Clinical and Laboratory Standards Institute (CLSI) Antimicrobial Susceptibility Testing Guidelines (CLSI-2010 and CLSI-2010-update) for Enterobacteriaceae in clinical microbiology laboratories in Taiwan. *Journal of*

Microbiology, Immunology and Infection, 43(5), 452-455.

Huang, H., Siehnel, R. J., Francis, B., Rawling, E., & Hancock, R. E. (1992). Analysis of two gene regions involved in the expression of the imipenem-specific, outer membrane porin protein OprD of Pseudomonas aeruginosa. *FEMS microbiology letters, 97*(3), 267-273.

Huang, X.-Z., Cash, D. M., Chahine, M. A., Nikolich, M. P., & Craft, D. W. (2012). Development and validation of a multiplex TaqMan real-time PCR for rapid detection of genes encoding four types of class D carbapenemase in Acinetobacter baumannii. *Journal of medical microbiology, 61*(11), 1532-1537.

Hugonnet, J.-E., Tremblay, L. W., Boshoff, H. I., Barry, C. E., & Blanchard, J. S. (2009). Meropenem-clavulanate is effective against extensively drug-resistant Mycobacterium tuberculosis. *Science, 323*(5918), 1215-1218.

Iacono, M., Villa, L., Fortini, D., Bordoni, R., Imperi, F., Bonnal, R. J., . . . Cassone, A. (2008). Whole-genome pyrosequencing of an epidemic multidrug-resistant Acinetobacter baumannii strain belonging to the European clone II group. *Antimicrobial agents and chemotherapy, 52*(7), 2616-2625.

Ilyas, M., Khurram, M., Ahmad, S., & Ahmad, I. (2015). Frequency, Susceptibility and Co-Existence of MBL, ESBL & AmpC Positive Pseudomonas aeruginosa in Tertiary Care Hospitals of Peshawar, KPK, Pakistan.

Irfan, S., Turton, J., Mehraj, J., Siddiqui, S., Haider, S., Zafar, A., . . . Hasan, R. (2011). Molecular and epidemiological characterisation of clinical isolates of carbapenem-resistant Acinetobacter baumannii from public and private sector intensive care units in Karachi, Pakistan. *Journal of Hospital Infection, 78*(2), 143-148.

Jeong, S. H., Bae, I. K., Kim, D., Hong, S. G., Song, J. S., Lee, J. H., & Lee, S. H. (2005). First outbreak of Klebsiella pneumoniae clinical isolates producing GES-5 and SHV-12 extended-spectrum β-lactamases in Korea. *Antimicrobial agents and chemotherapy, 49*(11), 4809-4810.

Johansson, Å., Ekelöf, J., Giske, C. G., & Sundqvist, M. (2014). The detection and verification of carbapenemases using ertapenem and Matrix Assisted Laser Desorption Ionization-Time of Flight. *BMC microbiology, 14*(1), 1.

Johnson, A. P., & Woodford, N. (2013). Global spread of antibiotic resistance: the example of New Delhi metallo-β-lactamase (NDM)-mediated carbapenem resistance. *Journal of medical microbiology, 62*(4), 499-513.

Jones, L. S., Toleman, M. A., Weeks, J. L., Howe, R. A., Walsh, T. R., & Kumarasamy, K. K. (2014). Plasmid carriage of blaNDM-1 in clinical Acinetobacter baumannii isolates from India. *Antimicrobial agents and chemotherapy, 58*(7), 4211-4213.

Jones, R. N., Deshpande, L., Fritsche, T. R., & Sader, H. S. (2004). Determination of epidemic clonality among multidrug-resistant strains of Acinetobacter spp. and Pseudomonas aeruginosa in the MYSTIC Programme (USA, 1999–2003). *Diagnostic microbiology and infectious disease, 49*(3), 211-216.

Kaase, M., Nordmann, P., Wichelhaus, T. A., Gatermann, S. G., Bonnin, R. A., & Poirel, L. (2011). NDM-2 carbapenemase in Acinetobacter baumannii from Egypt. *Journal of antimicrobial chemotherapy*, dkr135.

Kaase, M., Szabados, F., Anders, A., & Gatermann, S. G. (2014). Fosfomycin susceptibility in carbapenem-resistant Enterobacteriaceae from Germany. *Journal of clinical microbiology, 52*(6), 1893-1897.

Kaleem, F., Usman, J., Hassan, A., & Khan, A. (2010). Frequency and susceptibility pattern of metallo-beta-lactamase producers in a hospital in Pakistan. *The Journal of infection in developing countries, 4*(12), 810-813.

Kallen, M., Ricks, P., Edwards, J., MStat, A. S., Fridkin, S., Rasheed, J. K., . . . Patel, J. (2013). Vital signs: carbapenem-resistant Enterobacteriaceae. *MMWR Morb Mortal Wkly Rep, 62*, 165-170.

Kanj, S. S., & Kanafani, Z. A. (2011). *Current concepts in antimicrobial therapy against resistant gram-negative organisms: extended-spectrum β-lactamase–producing enterobacteriaceae, carbapenem-resistant enterobacteriaceae, and multidrug-resistant Pseudomonas aeruginosa.* Paper presented at the Mayo Clinic Proceedings.

Katayama, Y., Zhang, H.-Z., & Chambers, H. F. (2004). PBP 2a mutations producing very-high-level resistance to beta-lactams. *Antimicrobial agents and chemotherapy, 48*(2), 453-459.

Kim, J. Y., Jung, H. I., An, Y. J., Lee, J. H., Kim, S. J., Jeong, S. H., . . . Lee, S. H. (2006). Structural basis for the extended substrate spectrum of CMY-10, a plasmid-encoded class C β-lactamase. *Molecular microbiology, 60*(4), 907-916.

Koch-Weser, J., Sidel, V. W., Federman, E. B., Kanarek, P., Finer, D. C., & Eaton, A. E. (1970). Adverse Effects of Sodium ColistimethateManifestations and Specific Reaction Rates During 317 Courses of Therapy. *Annals of internal medicine, 72*(6), 857-868.

Koga, T., Sugihara, C., Kakuta, M., Masuda, N., Namba, E., & Fukuoka, T. (2009). Affinity of tomopenem (CS-023) for penicillin-binding proteins in Staphylococcus aureus, Escherichia coli, and Pseudomonas aeruginosa. *Antimicrobial agents and chemotherapy, 53*(3), 1238-1241.

Köhler, T., Michea-Hamzehpour, M., Epp, S. F., & Pechere, J.-C. (1999). Carbapenem activities against Pseudomonas aeruginosa: respective contributions of OprD and efflux systems. *Antimicrobial agents and chemotherapy, 43*(2), 424-427.

KONG, K. F., Schneper, L., & Mathee, K. (2010). Beta-lactam antibiotics: from antibiosis to resistance and bacteriology. *Apmis, 118*(1), 1-36.

Kotsanas, D., Wijesooriya, W., Korman, T. M., Gillespie, E. E., Wright, L., Snook, K., . . . Stuart, R. L. (2013). Down the drain": carbapenem-resistant bacteria in intensive care unit patients and handwashing sinks. *Med J Aust, 198*(5), 267-269.

Kumarasamy, K. K., Toleman, M. A., Walsh, T. R., Bagaria, J., Butt, F., Balakrishnan, R., . . . Irfan, S. (2010). Emergence of a new antibiotic resistance mechanism in India, Pakistan, and the UK: a molecular, biological, and epidemiological study. *The Lancet infectious diseases, 10*(9), 597-602.

Kunze, N., Moerer, O., Steinmetz, N., Schulze, M. H., Quintel, M., & Perl, T. (2015). Point-of-care multiplex PCR promises short turnaround times for microbial testing in hospital-acquired pneumonia–an observational pilot study in critical ill patients. *Annals of clinical microbiology and antimicrobials, 14*(1), 1.

Kurokawa, H., Yagi, T., Shibata, N., Shibayama, K., & Arakawa, Y.

(1999). Worldwide proliferation of carbapenem-resistant gram-negative bacteria. *The Lancet, 354*(9182), 955.

Landman, D., Salvani, J., Bratu, S., & Quale, J. (2005). Evaluation of techniques for detection of carbapenem-resistant Klebsiella pneumoniae in stool surveillance cultures. *Journal of clinical microbiology, 43*(11), 5639-5641.

Lange, C., Schubert, S., Jung, J., Kostrzewa, M., & Sparbier, K. (2014). Quantitative matrix-assisted laser desorption ionization–time of flight mass spectrometry for rapid resistance detection. *Journal of clinical microbiology, 52*(12), 4155-4162.

Laraki, N., Galleni, M., Thamm, I., Riccio, M. L., Amicosante, G., Frère, J.-M., & Rossolini, G. M. (1999). Structure of In31, abla IMP-containing Pseudomonas aeruginosa integron phyletically related to In5, which carries an unusual array of gene cassettes. *Antimicrobial agents and chemotherapy, 43*(4), 890-901.

Lascols, C., Hackel, M., Marshall, S. H., Hujer, A. M., Bouchillon, S., Badal, R., . . . Bonomo, R. A. (2011). Increasing prevalence and dissemination of NDM-1 metallo-β-lactamase in India: data from the SMART study (2009). *Journal of Antimicrobial Chemotherapy, 66*(9), 1992-1997.

Lauretti, L., Riccio, M. L., Mazzariol, A., Cornaglia, G., Amicosante, G., Fontana, R., & Rossolini, G. M. (1999). Cloning and characterization of bla VIM, a new integron-borne metallo-β-lactamase gene from a Pseudomonas aeruginosa clinical isolate. *Antimicrobial agents and chemotherapy, 43*(7), 1584-1590.

Ledeboer, N. A., Lopansri, B. K., Dhiman, N., Cavagnolo, R., Carroll, K. C., Granato, P., . . . Samuel, L. (2015). Identification of Gram-negative bacteria and genetic resistance determinants from positive blood culture broths by use of the Verigene Gram-negative blood culture multiplex microarray-based molecular assay. *Journal of clinical microbiology, 53*(8), 2460-2472.

Lee, C.-S. (2014). Therapy of infections due to carbapenem-resistant Gram-negative pathogens. *Infection & chemotherapy, 46*(3), 149-164.

Lee, E., Nicolas, M., Kitzis, M., Pialoux, G., Collatz, E., &

Gutmann, L. (1991). Association of two resistance mechanisms in a clinical isolate of Enterobacter cloacae with high-level resistance to imipenem. *Antimicrobial agents and chemotherapy, 35*(6), 1093-1098.

Lee, G. C., & Burgess, D. S. (2012). Treatment of Klebsiella pneumoniae carbapenemase (KPC) infections: a review of published case series and case reports. *Annals of clinical microbiology and antimicrobials, 11*(1), 32.

Lee, H.-Y., Chang, R.-C., Su, L.-H., Liu, S.-Y., Wu, S.-R., Chuang, C.-H., . . . Chiu, C.-H. (2012). Wide spread of Tn2006 in an AbaR4-type resistance island among carbapenem-resistant Acinetobacter baumannii clinical isolates in Taiwan. *International journal of antimicrobial agents, 40*(2), 163-167.

Lee, K., Lim, Y., Yong, D., Yum, J., & Chong, Y. (2003). Evaluation of the Hodge test and the imipenem-EDTA double-disk synergy test for differentiating metallo-β-lactamase-producing isolates of Pseudomonas spp. and Acinetobacter spp. *Journal of clinical microbiology, 41*(10), 4623-4629.

Lee, Y.-T., Huang, L.-Y., Chen, T.-L., Siu, L.-K., Fung, C.-P., Cho, W.-L., . . . Liu, C.-Y. (2009). Gene cassette arrays, antibiotic susceptibilities, and clinical characteristics of Acinetobacter baumannii bacteremic strains harboring class 1 integrons. *Journal of microbiology, immunology, and infection= Wei mian yu gan ran za zhi, 42*(3), 210-219.

Legaree, B. A., Daniels, K., Weadge, J. T., Cockburn, D., & Clarke, A. J. (2007). Function of penicillin-binding protein 2 in viability and morphology of Pseudomonas aeruginosa. *Journal of antimicrobial chemotherapy, 59*(3), 411-424.

Levy, S. B., & Marshall, B. (2004a). Antibacterial resistance worldwide: causes, challenges and responses. *Nature medicine, 10*(12s), S122.

Levy, S. B., & Marshall, B. (2004b). Antibacterial resistance worldwide: causes, challenges and responses. *Nature medicine, 10*, S122-S129.

Liao, X., & Hancock, R. (1997). Susceptibility to beta-lactam antibiotics of Pseudomonas aeruginosa overproducing penicillin-binding protein 3. *Antimicrobial agents and chemotherapy, 41*(5), 1158-1161.

Limansky, A. S., Mussi, M. A., & Viale, A. M. (2002). Loss of a 29-kilodalton outer membrane protein in Acinetobacter baumannii is associated with imipenem resistance. *Journal of clinical microbiology, 40*(12), 4776-4778.

Livermore, D. M. (2009). Has the era of untreatable infections arrived? *Journal of Antimicrobial Chemotherapy, 64*(suppl_1), i29-i36.

Livermore, D. M., Mushtaq, S., Warner, M., & Woodford, N. (2016). In-vitro activity of eravacycline against carbapenem-resistant Enterobacteriaceae and Acinetobacter baumannii. *Antimicrobial agents and chemotherapy*, AAC. 00436-00416.

Llanes, C., Hocquet, D., Vogne, C., Benali-Baitich, D., Neuwirth, C., & Plésiat, P. (2004). Clinical strains of Pseudomonas aeruginosa overproducing MexAB-OprM and MexXY efflux pumps simultaneously. *Antimicrobial agents and chemotherapy, 48*(5), 1797-1802.

Lodge, J., Minchin, S., Piddock, L., & Busby, S. (1990). Cloning, sequencing and analysis of the structural gene and regulatory region of the Pseudomonas aeruginosa chromosomal ampC β-lactamase. *Biochemical Journal, 272*(3), 627-631.

Lowe, C., Katz, K., McGeer, A., Muller, M. P., & Group, T. E. W. (2012). Disparity in infection control practices for multidrug-resistant Enterobacteriaceae. *American journal of infection control, 40*(9), 836-839.

Mahillon, J., & Chandler, M. (1998). Insertion sequences. *Microbiology and molecular biology reviews, 62*(3), 725-774.

Mainardi, J.-L., Mugnier, P., Coutrot, A., Buu-Hoi, A., Collatz, E., & Gutmann, L. (1997). Carbapenem resistance in a clinical isolate of Citrobacter freundii. *Antimicrobial agents and chemotherapy, 41*(11), 2352-2354.

Majiduddin, F. K., & Palzkill, T. (2005). Amino acid residues that contribute to substrate specificity of class A β-lactamase SME-1. *Antimicrobial agents and chemotherapy, 49*(8), 3421-3427.

Mammeri, H., Guillon, H., Eb, F., & Nordmann, P. (2010). Phenotypic and biochemical comparison of the carbapenem-hydrolyzing activities of five plasmid-borne

AmpC β-lactamases. *Antimicrobial agents and chemotherapy, 54*(11), 4556-4560.

Mao, W., Warren, M. S., Lee, A., Mistry, A., & Lomovskaya, O. (2001). MexXY-OprM efflux pump is required for antagonism of aminoglycosides by divalent cations inPseudomonas aeruginosa. *Antimicrobial agents and chemotherapy, 45*(7).

Marchaim, D., Navon-Venezia, S., Leavitt, A., Chmelnitsky, I., Schwaber, M. J., & Carmeli, Y. (2007). Molecular and epidemiologic study of polyclonal outbreaks of multidrug-resistant Acinetobacter baumannii infection in an Israeli hospital. *Infection Control & Hospital Epidemiology, 28*(8), 945-950.

Marshall, S., Hujer, A. M., Rojas, L. J., Papp-Wallace, K. M., Humphries, R. M., Spellberg, B., . . . Perez, F. (2017). Can ceftazidime-avibactam and aztreonam overcome β-lactam resistance conferred by metallo-β-lactamases in Enterobacteriaceae? *Antimicrobial Agents and Chemotherapy, 61*(4), e02243-02216.

Martí, S., Sánchez-Céspedes, J., Oliveira, E., Bellido, D., Giralt, E., & Vila, J. (2006). Proteomic analysis of a fraction enriched in cell envelope proteins of Acinetobacter baumannii. *Proteomics, 6*(S1).

Martínez-Martínez, L. (2008). Extended-spectrum β-lactamases and the permeability barrier. *Clinical Microbiology and Infection, 14*(s1), 82-89.

Maseda, H., Saito, K., Nakajima, A., & Nakae, T. (2000). Variation of the mexT gene, a regulator of the MexEF-oprN efflux pump expression in wild-type strains of Pseudomonas aeruginosa. *FEMS microbiology letters, 192*(1), 107-112.

Maseda, H., Sawada, I., Saito, K., Uchiyama, H., Nakae, T., & Nomura, N. (2004). Enhancement of the mexAB-oprM efflux pump expression by a quorum-sensing autoinducer and its cancellation by a regulator, MexT, of the mexEF-oprN efflux pump operon in Pseudomonas aeruginosa. *Antimicrobial agents and chemotherapy, 48*(4), 1320-1328.

Matsumoto, A., Hosoya, M., Kawasaki, Y., Katayose, M., Kato, K., & Suzuki, H. (2007). The emergence of drug-resistant Streptococcus pneumoniae and host risk factors for carriage of drug-resistant genes in northeastern Japan. *Japanese journal of infectious diseases, 60*(1), 10.

Maveyraud, L., Mourey, L., Kotra, L. P., Pedelacq, J.-D., Guillet, V., Mobashery, S., & Samama, J.-P. (1998). Structural basis for clinical longevity of carbapenem antibiotics in the face of challenge by the common class A β-lactamases from the antibiotic-resistant bacteria. *Journal of the American Chemical Society, 120*(38), 9748-9752.

Mazel, D. (2006). Integrons: agents of bacterial evolution. *Nature reviews. Microbiology, 4*(8), 608.

Mazel, D., Dychinco, B., Webb, V. A., & Davies, J. (1998). A distinctive class of integron in the Vibrio cholerae genome. *Science, 280*(5363), 605-608.

Meletis, G. (2016). Carbapenem resistance: overview of the problem and future perspectives. *Therapeutic advances in infectious disease, 3*(1), 15-21.

Meletis, G., Tzampaz, E., Protonotariou, E., & Sofianou, D. (2010). Emergence of Klebsiella pneumoniae carrying blaVIM and blaKPC genes. *Hippokratia, 14*(2), 139.

Mena, A., Plasencia, V., García, L., Hidalgo, O., Ayestarán, J. I., Alberti, S., . . . Oliver, A. (2006). Characterization of a large outbreak by CTX-M-1-producing Klebsiella pneumoniae and mechanisms leading to in vivo carbapenem resistance development. *Journal of clinical microbiology, 44*(8), 2831-2837.

Meric, M., Kasap, M., Gacar, G., Budak, F., Dundar, D., Kolayli, F., . . . Vahaboglu, H. (2008). Emergence and spread of carbapenem-resistant Acinetobacter baumannii in a tertiary care hospital in Turkey. *FEMS microbiology letters, 282*(2), 214-218.

Meroueh, S. O., Bencze, K. Z., Hesek, D., Lee, M., Fisher, J. F., Stemmler, T. L., & Mobashery, S. (2006). Three-dimensional structure of the bacterial cell wall peptidoglycan. *Proceedings of the National Academy of Sciences of the United States of America, 103*(12), 4404-4409.

Mine, T., Morita, Y., Kataoka, A., Mizushima, T., & Tsuchiya, T. (1999). Expression in Escherichia coli of a new multidrug efflux pump, MexXY, from Pseudomonas aeruginosa. *Antimicrobial Agents and Chemotherapy, 43*(2), 415-417.

Mingeot-Leclercq, M.-P., Glupczynski, Y., & Tulkens, P. M.

(1999). Aminoglycosides: activity and resistance. *Antimicrobial agents and chemotherapy, 43*(4), 727-737.

Mirande, C., Canard, I., Blanche, S. B. C., Charrier, J.-P., van Belkum, A., Welker, M., & Chatellier, S. (2015). Rapid detection of carbapenemase activity: benefits and weaknesses of MALDI-TOF MS. *European Journal of Clinical Microbiology & Infectious Diseases, 34*(11), 2225-2234.

Miriagou, V., Tzouvelekis, L. S., Rossiter, S., Tzelepi, E., Angulo, F. J., & Whichard, J. M. (2003). Imipenem resistance in a Salmonella clinical strain due to plasmid-mediated class A carbapenemase KPC-2. *Antimicrobial agents and chemotherapy, 47*(4), 1297-1300.

Misra, R., & Bavro, V. N. (2009). Assembly and transport mechanism of tripartite drug efflux systems. *Biochimica et Biophysica Acta (BBA)-Proteins and Proteomics, 1794*(5), 817-825.

Miyakis, S., Pefanis, A., & Tsakris, A. (2011). The challenges of antimicrobial drug resistance in Greece. *Clinical infectious diseases, 53*(2), 177-184.

Moellering, R. C., Eliopoulos, G. M., & Sentochnik, D. E. (1989). The carbapenems: new broad spectrum β-lactam antibiotics. *Journal of antimicrobial chemotherapy, 24*(suppl A), 1-7.

Morrill, H. J., Pogue, J. M., Kaye, K. S., & LaPlante, K. L. (2015a). *Treatment options for carbapenem-resistant Enterobacteriaceae infections.* Paper presented at the Open forum infectious diseases.

Morrill, H. J., Pogue, J. M., Kaye, K. S., & LaPlante, K. L. (2015b). *Treatment options for carbapenem-resistant Enterobacteriaceae infections.* Paper presented at the Open forum infectious diseases.

Mugnier, P., Poirel, L., Pitout, M., & Nordmann, P. (2008). Carbapenem-resistant and OXA-23-producing Acinetobacter baumannii isolates in the United Arab Emirates. *Clinical Microbiology and Infection, 14*(9), 879-882.

Munoz-Price, L. S., Poirel, L., Bonomo, R. A., Schwaber, M. J., Daikos, G. L., Cormican, M., . . . Hayden, M. K. (2013). Clinical epidemiology of the global expansion of Klebsiella pneumoniae carbapenemases. *The Lancet infectious diseases,*

13(9), 785-796.
Mussi, M. A., Limansky, A. S., & Viale, A. M. (2005). Acquisition of resistance to carbapenems in multidrug-resistant clinical strains of Acinetobacter baumannii: natural insertional inactivation of a gene encoding a member of a novel family of β-barrel outer membrane proteins. *Antimicrobial agents and chemotherapy, 49*(4), 1432-1440.
Naas, T., & Nordmann, P. (1994). Analysis of a carbapenem-hydrolyzing class A beta-lactamase from Enterobacter cloacae and of its LysR-type regulatory protein. *Proceedings of the National Academy of Sciences, 91*(16), 7693-7697.
Naas, T., Vandel, L., Sougakoff, W., Livermore, D. M., & Nordmann, P. (1994). Cloning and sequence analysis of the gene for a carbapenem-hydrolyzing class A beta-lactamase, Sme-1, from Serratia marcescens S6. *Antimicrobial Agents and Chemotherapy, 38*(6), 1262-1270.
Nahid, F., Khan, A. A., Rehman, S., & Zahra, R. (2013). Prevalence of metallo-β-lactamase NDM-1-producing multi-drug resistant bacteria at two Pakistani hospitals and implications for public health. *Journal of infection and public health, 6*(6), 487-493.
Neuwirth, C., Siébor, E., Duez, J.-M., Péchinot, A., & Kazmierczak, A. (1995). Imipenem resistance in clinical isolates of Proteus mirabilis associated with alterations in penicillin-binding proteins. *Journal of Antimicrobial Chemotherapy, 36*(2), 335-342.
Nikaido, H. (1996). Multidrug efflux pumps of gram-negative bacteria. *Journal of bacteriology, 178*(20), 5853.
Nikaido, H. (2003). Molecular basis of bacterial outer membrane permeability revisited. *Microbiology and molecular biology reviews, 67*(4), 593-656.
Nitzan, Y., Pechatnikov, I., Bar-El, D., & Wexler, H. (1999). Isolation and characterization of heat-modifiable proteins from the outer membrane of Porphyromonas asaccharolytica and Acinetobacter baumannii. *Anaerobe, 5*(1), 43-50.
Nix, D. E., Majumdar, A. K., & DiNubile, M. J. (2004). Pharmacokinetics and pharmacodynamics of ertapenem: an overview for clinicians. *Journal of Antimicrobial Chemotherapy,*

53(suppl_2), ii23-ii28.
Nordmann, P. (1998). Trends in β-lactam resistance among Enterobacteriaceae. *Clinical infectious diseases, 27*(Supplement_1), S100-S106.
Nordmann, P., Naas, T., & Poirel, L. (2011). Global spread of carbapenemase-producing Enterobacteriaceae. *Emerging infectious diseases, 17*(10), 1791.
Nordmann, P., Picazo, J. J., Mutters, R., Korten, V., Quintana, A., Laeuffer, J. M., . . . Group, C. S. (2011). Comparative activity of carbapenem testing: the COMPACT study. *Journal of antimicrobial chemotherapy, 66*(5), 1070-1078.
Nordmann, P., & Poirel, L. (2002). Emerging carbapenemases in Gram-negative aerobes. *Clinical microbiology and infection, 8*(6), 321-331.
NOZAKI, Y., HARADA, S., KITANO, K., & IMADA, A. (1984). Structure-activity relations of 5, 6-cis carbapenem antibiotics and role of factors determining susceptibility of Escherichia coli to β-lactam antibiotics. *The Journal of antibiotics, 37*(3), 218-226.
Obara, M., & Nakae, T. (1991). Mechanisms of resistance to β-lactam antibiotics in Acinetobacter calcoaceticus. *Journal of Antimicrobial Chemotherapy, 28*(6), 791-800.
Ochs, M. M., McCusker, M. P., Bains, M., & Hancock, R. E. (1999). Negative regulation of the Pseudomonas aeruginosa outer membrane porin OprD selective for imipenem and basic amino acids. *Antimicrobial agents and chemotherapy, 43*(5), 1085-1090.
Olaitan, A. O., Morand, S., & Rolain, J.-M. (2014). Mechanisms of polymyxin resistance: acquired and intrinsic resistance in bacteria. *Frontiers in microbiology, 5*, 643.
Oliver, A., Levin, B. R., Juan, C., Baquero, F., & Blázquez, J. (2004). Hypermutation and the preexistence of antibiotic-resistant Pseudomonas aeruginosa mutants: implications for susceptibility testing and treatment of chronic infections. *Antimicrobial agents and chemotherapy, 48*(11), 4226-4233.
Osaki, Y., Sanbongi, Y., Ishikawa, M., Kataoka, H., Suzuki, T., Maeda, K., & Ida, T. (2005). Genetic approach to study the relationship between penicillin-binding protein 3 mutations

and Haemophilus influenzae β-lactam resistance by using site-directed mutagenesis and gene recombinants. *Antimicrobial agents and chemotherapy, 49*(7), 2834-2839.

Österblad, M., Hakanen, A. J., & Jalava, J. (2014). Evaluation of the Carba NP test for carbapenemase detection. *Antimicrobial agents and chemotherapy, 58*(12), 7553-7556.

Oteo, J., Hernández-Almaraz, J. L., Gil-Antón, J., Vindel, A., Fernández, S., Bautista, V., & Campos, J. (2010). Outbreak of vim-1-carbapenemase-producing Enterobacter cloacae in a pediatric intensive care unit. *The Pediatric infectious disease journal, 29*(12), 1144-1146.

Pai, H., Kim, J.-W., Kim, J., Lee, J. H., Choe, K. W., & Gotoh, N. (2001). Carbapenem resistance mechanisms in Pseudomonas aeruginosa clinical isolates. *Antimicrobial agents and chemotherapy, 45*(2), 480-484.

Palzkill, T. (2013). Metallo-β-lactamase structure and function. *Annals of the New York Academy of Sciences, 1277*(1), 91-104.

Pang, Y., Lu, J., Wang, Y., Song, Y., Wang, S., & Zhao, Y. (2013). Study of the rifampin monoresistance mechanism in Mycobacterium tuberculosis. *Antimicrobial agents and chemotherapy, 57*(2), 893-900.

Papagiannitsis, C. C., Giakkoupi, P., Vatopoulos, A. C., Tryfinopoulou, K., Miriagou, V., & Tzouvelekis, L. S. (2010). Emergence of Klebsiella pneumoniae of a novel sequence type (ST383) producing VIM-4, KPC-2 and CMY-4 β-lactamases. *International journal of antimicrobial agents, 36*(6), 573-574.

Papp-Wallace, K. M., Endimiani, A., Taracila, M. A., & Bonomo, R. A. (2011). Carbapenems: past, present, and future. *Antimicrobial agents and chemotherapy, 55*(11), 4943-4960.

Papp-Wallace, K. M., Taracila, M., Hornick, J. M., Hujer, A. M., Hujer, K. M., Distler, A. M., . . . Bonomo, R. A. (2010). Substrate selectivity and a novel role in inhibitor discrimination by residue 237 in the KPC-2 β-lactamase. *Antimicrobial agents and chemotherapy, 54*(7), 2867-2877.

Papp-Wallace, K. M., Taracila, M., Wallace, C. J., Hujer, K. M., Bethel, C. R., Hornick, J. M., & Bonomo, R. A. (2010). Elucidating the role of Trp105 in the KPC-2 β-lactamase. *Protein Science, 19*(9), 1714-1727.

Paul, M., Carmeli, Y., Durante-Mangoni, E., Mouton, J. W., Tacconelli, E., Theuretzbacher, U., . . . Leibovici, L. (2014). Combination therapy for carbapenem-resistant Gram-negative bacteria. *Journal of Antimicrobial Chemotherapy*, dku168.

Peleg, A. Y., Franklin, C., Bell, J. M., & Spelman, D. W. (2005). Dissemination of the metallo-β-lactamase gene blaIMP-4 among gram-negative pathogens in a clinical setting in Australia. *Clinical Infectious Diseases, 41*(11), 1549-1556.

Peleg, A. Y., Seifert, H., & Paterson, D. L. (2008). Acinetobacter baumannii: emergence of a successful pathogen. *Clinical microbiology reviews, 21*(3), 538-582.

Perron, K., Caille, O., Rossier, C., van Delden, C., Dumas, J.-L., & Köhler, T. (2004). CzcR-CzcS, a two-component system involved in heavy metal and carbapenem resistance in Pseudomonas aeruginosa. *Journal of Biological Chemistry, 279*(10), 8761-8768.

Piddock, L., & Jin, Y. (1995). Activity of biapenem (LJC 10627) against 51 imipenem-resistant bacteria and selection and characterisation of biapenem-resistant mutants. *Journal of Antimicrobial Chemotherapy, 36*(5), 845-850.

Pierre, J., Boisivon, A., & Gutmann, L. (1990). Alteration of PBP 3 entails resistance to imipenem in Listeria monocytogenes. *Antimicrobial agents and chemotherapy, 34*(9), 1695-1698.

Pitout, J. D., & Laupland, K. B. (2008). Extended-spectrum β-lactamase-producing Enterobacteriaceae: an emerging public-health concern. *The Lancet infectious diseases, 8*(3), 159-166.

Poirel, L., Figueiredo, S., Cattoir, V., Carattoli, A., & Nordmann, P. (2008). Acinetobacter radioresistens as a silent source of carbapenem resistance for Acinetobacter spp. *Antimicrobial agents and chemotherapy, 52*(4), 1252-1256.

Poirel, L., Héritier, C., Spicq, C., & Nordmann, P. (2004). In vivo acquisition of high-level resistance to imipenem in Escherichia coli. *Journal of clinical microbiology, 42*(8), 3831-3833.

Poirel, L., Le Thomas, I., Naas, T., Karim, A., & Nordmann, P. (2000). Biochemical sequence analyses of GES-1, a novel class A extended-spectrum β-lactamase, and the class 1 integron In52 from Klebsiella pneumoniae. *Antimicrobial agents and chemotherapy, 44*(3), 622-632.

Poirel, L., Mansour, W., Bouallegue, O., & Nordmann, P. (2008). Carbapenem-resistant Acinetobacter baumannii isolates from Tunisia producing the OXA-58-like carbapenem-hydrolyzing oxacillinase OXA-97. *Antimicrobial agents and chemotherapy, 52*(5), 1613-1617.

Poirel, L., Marqué, S., Héritier, C., Segonds, C., Chabanon, G., & Nordmann, P. (2005). OXA-58, a novel class D β-lactamase involved in resistance to carbapenems in Acinetobacter baumannii. *Antimicrobial agents and chemotherapy, 49*(1), 202-208.

Poirel, L., Naas, T., Nicolas, D., Collet, L., Bellais, S., Cavallo, J.-D., & Nordmann, P. (2000). Characterization of VIM-2, a carbapenem-hydrolyzing metallo-β-lactamase and its plasmid-and integron-borne gene from a Pseudomonas aeruginosa clinical isolate in France. *Antimicrobial agents and chemotherapy, 44*(4), 891-897.

Poirel, L., Naas, T., & Nordmann, P. (2010). Diversity, epidemiology, and genetics of class D β-lactamases. *Antimicrobial agents and chemotherapy, 54*(1), 24-38.

Poirel, L., & Nordmann, P. (2002). Acquired carbapenem-hydrolyzing beta-lactamases and their genetic support. *Current pharmaceutical biotechnology, 3*(2), 117-127.

Poirel, L., & Nordmann, P. (2006). Carbapenem resistance in Acinetobacter baumannii: mechanisms and epidemiology. *Clinical Microbiology and Infection, 12*(9), 826-836.

Poirel, L., Pitout, J. D., & Nordmann, P. (2007). Carbapenemases: molecular diversity and clinical consequences. *Future Microbiology, 2*(5), 501-512.

Poirel, L., Walsh, T. R., Cuvillier, V., & Nordmann, P. (2011). Multiplex PCR for detection of acquired carbapenemase genes. *Diagnostic microbiology and infectious disease, 70*(1), 119-123.

Poirel, L., Weldhagen, G. F., Naas, T., De Champs, C., Dove, M. G., & Nordmann, P. (2001). GES-2, a Class A β-Lactamase fromPseudomonas aeruginosa with Increased Hydrolysis of Imipenem. *Antimicrobial agents and chemotherapy, 45*(9), 2598-2603.

Pollitt, S., & Zalkin, H. (1983). Role of primary structure and disulfide bond formation in beta-lactamase secretion. *Journal of bacteriology*, *153*(1), 27-32.

Poole, K. (2002). Outer membranes and efflux: the path to multidrug resistance in Gram-negative bacteria. *Current pharmaceutical biotechnology*, *3*(2), 77-98.

Poole, K., Tetro, K., Zhao, Q., Neshat, S., Heinrichs, D. E., & Bianco, N. (1996). Expression of the multidrug resistance operon mexA-mexB-oprM in Pseudomonas aeruginosa: mexR encodes a regulator of operon expression. *Antimicrobial Agents and Chemotherapy*, *40*(9), 2021-2028.

Post, V., White, P. A., & Hall, R. M. (2010). Evolution of AbaR-type genomic resistance islands in multiply antibiotic-resistant Acinetobacter baumannii. *Journal of Antimicrobial Chemotherapy*, *65*(6), 1162-1170.

Pournaras, S., Maniati, M., Petinaki, E., Tzouvelekis, L., Tsakris, A., Legakis, N., & Maniatis, A. (2003). Hospital outbreak of multiple clones of Pseudomonas aeruginosa carrying the unrelated metallo-β-lactamase gene variants blaVIM-2 and blaVIM-4. *Journal of antimicrobial chemotherapy*, *51*(6), 1409-1414.

Pournaras, S., Maniati, M., Spanakis, N., Ikonomidis, A., Tassios, P., Tsakris, A., . . . Maniatis, A. (2005). Spread of efflux pump-overexpressing, non-metallo-β-lactamase-producing, meropenem-resistant but ceftazidime-susceptible Pseudomonas aeruginosa in a region with blaVIM endemicity. *Journal of Antimicrobial Chemotherapy*, *56*(4), 761-764.

Pournaras, S., Markogiannakis, A., Ikonomidis, A., Kondyli, L., Bethimouti, K., Maniatis, A., . . . Tsakris, A. (2006). Outbreak of multiple clones of imipenem-resistant Acinetobacter baumannii isolates expressing OXA-58 carbapenemase in an intensive care unit. *Journal of Antimicrobial Chemotherapy*, *57*(3), 557-561.

Pournaras, S., Zarkotou, O., Poulou, A., Kristo, I., Vrioni, G., Themeli-Digalaki, K., & Tsakris, A. (2013). A combined disk test for direct differentiation of carbapenemase-producing Enterobacteriaceae in surveillance rectal swabs. *Journal of clinical microbiology*, *51*(9), 2986-2990.

Pulido, M. R., García-Quintanilla, M., Martín-Peña, R., Cisneros, J. M., & McConnell, M. J. (2013). Progress on the development of rapid methods for antimicrobial susceptibility testing. *Journal of Antimicrobial Chemotherapy*, dkt253.

Quale, J., Bratu, S., Gupta, J., & Landman, D. (2006). Interplay of efflux system, ampC, and oprD expression in carbapenem resistance of Pseudomonas aeruginosa clinical isolates. *Antimicrobial agents and chemotherapy, 50*(5), 1633-1641.

Queenan, A. M., & Bush, K. (2007). Carbapenemases: the versatile β-lactamases. *Clinical microbiology reviews, 20*(3), 440-458.

Queenan, A. M., Shang, W., Flamm, R., & Bush, K. (2010). Hydrolysis and inhibition profiles of β-lactamases from molecular classes A to D with doripenem, imipenem, and meropenem. *Antimicrobial agents and chemotherapy, 54*(1), 565-569.

Rai, S., Manchanda, V., Singh, N., & Kaur, I. (2011). Zinc-dependent carbapenemases in clinical isolates of family Enterobacteriaceae. *Indian Journal of medical microbiology, 29*(3), 275.

Raimondi, A., Traverso, A., & Nikaido, H. (1991). Imipenem-and meropenem-resistant mutants of Enterobacter cloacae and Proteus rettgeri lack porins. *Antimicrobial agents and chemotherapy, 35*(6), 1174-1180.

Raquet, X., Lamotte-Brasseur, J., Bouillenne, F., & Frère, J. M. (1997). A disulfide bridge near the active site of carbapenem-hydrolyzing class A β-lactamases might explain their unusual substrate profile. *Proteins: Structure, Function, and Bioinformatics, 27*(1), 47-58.

Ravasi, P., Limansky, A. S., Rodriguez, R. E., Viale, A. M., & Mussi, M. A. (2011). ISAba825, a functional insertion sequence modulating genomic plasticity and blaOXA-58 expression in Acinetobacter baumannii. *Antimicrobial agents and chemotherapy, 55*(2), 917-920.

Rhomberg, P. R., & Jones, R. N. (2009). Summary trends for the meropenem yearly susceptibility test information collection program: a 10-year experience in the United States (1999–2008). *Diagnostic microbiology and infectious disease, 65*(4), 414-426.

Riccio, M. L., Franceschini, N., Boschi, L., Caravelli, B., Cornaglia, G., Fontana, R., . . . Rossolini, G. M. (2000). Characterization of the metallo-β-lactamase determinant of Acinetobacter baumannii AC-54/97 reveals the existence of bla IMP allelic variants carried by gene cassettes of different phylogeny. *Antimicrobial agents and chemotherapy, 44*(5), 1229-1235.

Riera, E., Cabot, G., Mulet, X., García-Castillo, M., del Campo, R., Juan, C., . . . Oliver, A. (2011). Pseudomonas aeruginosa carbapenem resistance mechanisms in Spain: impact on the activity of imipenem, meropenem and doripenem. *Journal of antimicrobial chemotherapy, 66*(9), 2022-2027.

Rödel, J., Karrasch, M., Edel, B., Stoll, S., Bohnert, J., Löffler, B., . . . Pfister, W. (2016). Antibiotic treatment algorithm development based on a microarray nucleic acid assay for rapid bacterial identification and resistance determination from positive blood cultures. *Diagnostic microbiology and infectious disease, 84*(3), 252-257.

Rodloff, A., Goldstein, E., & Torres, A. (2006). Two decades of imipenem therapy. *Journal of Antimicrobial Chemotherapy, 58*(5), 916-929.

Rodríguez-Martínez, J.-M., Poirel, L., & Nordmann, P. (2009a). Extended-spectrum cephalosporinases in Pseudomonas aeruginosa. *Antimicrobial agents and chemotherapy, 53*(5), 1766-1771.

Rodríguez-Martínez, J.-M., Poirel, L., & Nordmann, P. (2009b). Molecular epidemiology and mechanisms of carbapenem resistance in Pseudomonas aeruginosa. *Antimicrobial agents and chemotherapy, 53*(11), 4783-4788.

Saito, K., Akama, H., Yoshihara, E., & Nakae, T. (2003). Mutations affecting DNA-binding activity of the MexR repressor of mexR-mexA-mexB-oprM operon expression. *Journal of bacteriology, 185*(20), 6195-6198.

Saito, K., Yoneyama, H., & Nakae, T. (1999). nalB-type mutations causing the overexpression of the MexAB-OprM efflux pump are located in the mexR gene of the Pseudomonas aeruginosa chromosome. *FEMS microbiology letters, 179*(1), 67-72.

Sato, K., & Nakae, T. (1991). Outer membrane permeability of

Acinetobacter calcoaceticus and its implication in antibiotic resistance. *Journal of Antimicrobial Chemotherapy, 28*(1), 35-45.

Sauvage, E., Kerff, F., Terrak, M., Ayala, J. A., & Charlier, P. (2008). The penicillin-binding proteins: structure and role in peptidoglycan biosynthesis. *FEMS microbiology reviews, 32*(2), 234-258.

Schmidt, H., & Hensel, M. (2004). Pathogenicity islands in bacterial pathogenesis. *Clinical microbiology reviews, 17*(1), 14-56.

Senda, K., Arakawa, Y., Nakashima, K., Ito, H., Ichiyama, S., Shimokata, K., . . . Ohta, M. (1996). Multifocal outbreaks of metallo-beta-lactamase-producing Pseudomonas aeruginosa resistant to broad-spectrum beta-lactams, including carbapenems. *Antimicrobial agents and chemotherapy, 40*(2), 349-353.

Shan, S., Sajid, S., & Ahmad, K. (2015). Detection of bla IMP Gene in Metallo-β-Lactamase Producing Isolates of Imipenem Resistant Pseudomonas aeruginosa; an Alarming Threat. *Journal of Microbiology Research, 5*(6), 175-180.

Sharma, A., Bakthavatchalam, Y. D., Gopi, R., An, S., Verghese, V. P., & Veeraraghavan, B. (2016). Mechanisms of Carbapenem Resistance in K. pneumoniae and E. coli from Bloodstream Infections in India. *Journal of Infectious Diseases & Therapy*.

Shukla, I., Tiwari, R., & Agrawal, M. (2004). Prevalence of extended spectrum-lactamase producing Klebsiella pneumoniae in a tertiary care hospital. *Indian journal of medical microbiology, 22*(2), 87.

Siegel, J., & Rhinehart, E. (2007). Health Care Infection Control Practices Advisory Committee. 2007 Guideline for isolation precautions: preventing transmission of infectious agents in health care settings.

Sievert, D. M., Ricks, P., Edwards, J. R., Schneider, A., Patel, J., Srinivasan, A., . . . Fridkin, S. (2013). Antimicrobial-resistant pathogens associated with healthcare-associated infections summary of data reported to the National Healthcare Safety Network at the Centers for Disease Control and Prevention, 2009–2010. *Infection Control & Hospital Epidemiology, 34*(01), 1-14.

Siroy, A., Molle, V., Lemaître-Guillier, C., Vallenet, D., Pestel-Caron, M., Cozzone, A. J., ... Dé, E. (2005). Channel formation by CarO, the carbapenem resistance-associated outer membrane protein of Acinetobacter baumannii. *Antimicrobial agents and chemotherapy, 49*(12), 4876-4883.

Smith Moland, E., Hanson, N. D., Herrera, V. L., Black, J. A., Lockhart, T. J., Hossain, A., ... Thomson, K. S. (2003). Plasmid-mediated, carbapenem-hydrolysing β-lactamase, KPC-2, in Klebsiella pneumoniae isolates. *Journal of Antimicrobial Chemotherapy, 51*(3), 711-714.

Sobel, M. L., McKay, G. A., & Poole, K. (2003). Contribution of the MexXY multidrug transporter to aminoglycoside resistance in Pseudomonas aeruginosa clinical isolates. *Antimicrobial agents and chemotherapy, 47*(10), 3202-3207.

Song, J., Xie, G., Elf, P. K., Young, K. D., & Jensen, R. A. (1998). Comparative analysis of Pseudomonas aeruginosa penicillin-binding protein 7 in the context of its membership in the family of low-molecular-mass PBPs. *Microbiology, 144*(4), 975-983.

Sood, S. (2016). Chloramphenicol–A Potent Armament Against Multi-Drug Resistant (MDR) Gram Negative Bacilli? *Journal of clinical and diagnostic research: JCDR, 10*(2), DC01.

Srikumar, R., Paul, C. J., & Poole, K. (2000). Influence of mutations in the mexR repressor gene on expression of the MexA-MexB-oprM multidrug efflux system ofPseudomonas aeruginosa. *Journal of Bacteriology, 182*(5), 1410-1414.

Stapleton, P. D., Shannon, K. P., & French, G. L. (1999). Carbapenem resistance in Escherichia coli associated with plasmid-determined CMY-4 β-lactamase production and loss of an outer membrane protein. *Antimicrobial agents and chemotherapy, 43*(5), 1206-1210.

Stokes, H. T., & Hall, R. M. (1989). A novel family of potentially mobile DNA elements encoding site-specific gene-integration functions: integrons. *Molecular microbiology, 3*(12), 1669-1683.

Sumita, Y., & Fakasawa, M. (1995). Potent activity of meropenem against Escherichia coli arising from its simultaneous binding to penicillin-binding proteins 2 and 3. *Journal of*

Antimicrobial Chemotherapy, 36(1), 53-64.

Symmons, M. F., Bokma, E., Koronakis, E., Hughes, C., & Koronakis, V. (2009). The assembled structure of a complete tripartite bacterial multidrug efflux pump. *Proceedings of the National Academy of Sciences, 106*(17), 7173-7178.

Tamber, S., & Hancock, R. E. (2006). Involvement of two related porins, OprD and OpdP, in the uptake of arginine by Pseudomonas aeruginosa. *FEMS microbiology letters, 260*(1), 23-29.

Tamma, P. D., Cosgrove, S. E., & Maragakis, L. L. (2012). Combination therapy for treatment of infections with gram-negative bacteria. *Clinical microbiology reviews, 25*(3), 450-470.

Taneja, N., & Kaur, H. (2016). Insights into newer antimicrobial agents against gram-negative bacteria. *Microbiology insights, 9*, 9.

Tato, M., Ruiz-Garbajosa, P., Traczewski, M., Dodgson, A., McEwan, A., Humphries, R., . . . Cantón, R. (2016). Multisite evaluation of Cepheid Xpert-Carba-R Assay for the detection of carbapenemase-producing organisms in rectal swabs. *Journal of clinical microbiology*, JCM. 00341-00316.

Thomson, K. S. (2010). Extended-spectrum-β-lactamase, AmpC, and carbapenemase issues. *Journal of clinical microbiology, 48*(4), 1019-1025.

Tipper, D. J., & Strominger, J. L. (1965). Mechanism of action of penicillins: a proposal based on their structural similarity to acyl-D-alanyl-D-alanine. *Proceedings of the National Academy of Sciences, 54*(4), 1133-1141.

Toleman, M. A., Rolston, K., Jones, R. N., & Walsh, T. R. (2004). blaVIM-7, an evolutionarily distinct metallo-β-lactamase gene in a Pseudomonas aeruginosa isolate from the United States. *Antimicrobial agents and chemotherapy, 48*(1), 329-332.

Toleman, M. A., Simm, A. M., Murphy, T. A., Gales, A. C., Biedenbach, D. J., Jones, R. N., & Walsh, T. R. (2002). Molecular characterization of SPM-1, a novel metallo-β-lactamase isolated in Latin America: report from the SENTRY antimicrobial surveillance programme. *Journal of antimicrobial chemotherapy, 50*(5), 673-679.

Tsakris, A., Kristo, I., Vrioni, G., Themeli-Digalaki, K., Pournaras, S., Zarkotou, O., & Poulou, A. (2013). A Combined Disk Test for Direct.

Tumbarello, M., Viale, P., Viscoli, C., Trecarichi, E. M., Tumietto, F., Marchese, A., . . . Cristini, F. (2012). Predictors of mortality in bloodstream infections caused by Klebsiella pneumoniae carbapenemase–producing K. pneumoniae: importance of combination therapy. *Clinical Infectious Diseases, 55*(7), 943-950.

Vaidya, V. K. (2011). Horizontal transfer of antimicrobial resistance by extended-spectrum β lactamase-producing enterobacteriaceae. *Journal of laboratory physicians, 3*(1), 37.

van Belkum, A., & Dunne, W. M. (2013). Next-generation antimicrobial susceptibility testing. *Journal of clinical microbiology, 51*(7), 2018-2024.

Vila, J. (1998). Mechanisms of antimicrobial resistance in Acinetobacter baumannii. *Reviews in Medical Microbiology, 9*(2), 87-98.

Vila, J., Martí, S., & Sánchez-Céspedes, J. (2007). Porins, efflux pumps and multidrug resistance in Acinetobacter baumannii. *Journal of Antimicrobial Chemotherapy, 59*(6), 1210-1215.

Villalón, P., Valdezate, S., Medina-Pascual, M. J., Carrasco, G., Vindel, A., & Saez-Nieto, J. A. (2012). Epidemiology of the Acinetobacter-derived cephalosporinase, carbapenem-hydrolysing oxacillinase and metallo-β-lactamase genes, and of common insertion sequences, in epidemic clones of Acinetobacter baumannii from Spain. *Journal of Antimicrobial Chemotherapy, 68*(3), 550-553.

Villegas, M. V., Lolans, K., Correa, A., Kattan, J. N., Lopez, J. A., Quinn, J. P., & Group, C. N. R. S. (2007). First identification of Pseudomonas aeruginosa isolates producing a KPC-type carbapenem-hydrolyzing β-lactamase. *Antimicrobial agents and chemotherapy, 51*(4), 1553-1555.

Villegas, M. V., Lolans, K., Correa, A., Suarez, C. J., Lopez, J. A., Vallejo, M., . . . Group, C. N. R. S. (2006). First detection of the plasmid-mediated class A carbapenemase KPC-2 in clinical isolates of Klebsiella pneumoniae from South America. *Antimicrobial agents and chemotherapy, 50*(8), 2880-2882.

Vogne, C., Aires, J. R., Bailly, C., Hocquet, D., & Plésiat, P. (2004). Role of the multidrug efflux system MexXY in the emergence of moderate resistance to aminoglycosides among Pseudomonas aeruginosa isolates from patients with cystic fibrosis. *Antimicrobial agents and chemotherapy, 48*(5), 1676-1680.

Walsh, T. R. (2008). Clinically significant carbapenemases: an update. *Current opinion in infectious diseases, 21*(4), 367-371.

Walsh, T. R. (2010). Emerging carbapenemases: a global perspective. *International journal of antimicrobial agents, 36*, S8-S14.

Walsh, T. R., Toleman, M. A., Poirel, L., & Nordmann, P. (2005). Metallo-β-lactamases: the quiet before the storm? *Clinical microbiology reviews, 18*(2), 306-325.

Walther-Rasmussen, J., & Høiby, N. (2006). OXA-type carbapenemases. *Journal of antimicrobial chemotherapy, 57*(3), 373-383.

Walther-Rasmussen, J., & Høiby, N. (2007). Class A carbapenemases. *Journal of antimicrobial chemotherapy, 60*(3), 470-482.

Wang, J., Zhou, J.-y., Qu, T.-t., Shen, P., Wei, Z.-q., Yu, Y.-s., & Li, L.-j. (2010). Molecular epidemiology and mechanisms of carbapenem resistance in Pseudomonas aeruginosa isolates from Chinese hospitals. *International journal of antimicrobial agents, 35*(5), 486-491.

Wareham, D. W., & Bean, D. C. (2006). In-vitro activity of polymyxin B in combination with imipenem, rifampicin and azithromycin versus multidrug resistant strains of Acinetobacter baumannii producing OXA-23 carbapenemases. *Annals of clinical microbiology and antimicrobials, 5*(1), 10.

Weiss, D. S., Chen, J. C., Ghigo, J.-M., Boyd, D., & Beckwith, J. (1999). Localization of FtsI (PBP3) to the septal ring requires its membrane anchor, the Z ring, FtsA, FtsQ, and FtsL. *Journal of bacteriology, 181*(2), 508-520.

White, P. A., McIver, C. J., & Rawlinson, W. D. (2001). Integrons and gene cassettes in theenterobacteriaceae. *Antimicrobial agents and chemotherapy, 45*(9), 2658-2661.

Wolter, D. J., Smith-Moland, E., Goering, R. V., Hanson, N. D., & Lister, P. D. (2004). Multidrug resistance associated with mexXY expression in clinical isolates of Pseudomonas aeruginosa from a Texas hospital. *Diagnostic microbiology and infectious disease, 50*(1), 43-50.

Wood, G. C., Hanes, S. D., Boucher, B. A., Croce, M. A., & Fabian, T. C. (2003). Tetracyclines for treating multidrug-resistant Acinetobacter baumannii ventilator-associated pneumonia. *Intensive care medicine, 29*(11), 2072-2076.

Woodford, N., & Johnson, A. P. (2004). *Genomics, proteomics, and clinical bacteriology*: Springer.

Wu, S., Xu, D., & Guo, H. (2010). QM/MM studies of monozinc β-lactamase CphA suggest that the crystal structure of an enzyme− intermediate complex represents a minor pathway. *Journal of the American Chemical Society, 132*(51), 17986-17988.

Xu, D., Xie, D., & Guo, H. (2006). Catalytic mechanism of class B2 metallo-β-lactamase. *Journal of Biological Chemistry, 281*(13), 8740-8747.

Yigit, H., Queenan, A. M., Anderson, G. J., Domenech-Sanchez, A., Biddle, J. W., Steward, C. D., . . . Tenover, F. C. (2001). Novel carbapenem-hydrolyzing β-lactamase, KPC-1, from a carbapenem-resistant strain of Klebsiella pneumoniae. *Antimicrobial agents and chemotherapy, 45*(4), 1151-1161.

Yigit, H., Queenan, A. M., Rasheed, J. K., Biddle, J. W., Domenech-Sanchez, A., Alberti, S., . . . Tenover, F. C. (2003). Carbapenem-resistant strain of Klebsiella oxytoca harboring carbapenem-hydrolyzingβ-lactamase KPC-2. *Antimicrobial agents and chemotherapy, 47*(12), 3881-3889.

Yoneyama, H., Ocaktan, A., Tsuda, M., & Nakae, T. (1997). The Role ofmex-Gene Products in Antibiotic Extrusion inPseudomonas aeruginosa. *Biochemical and biophysical research communications, 233*(3), 611-618.

Yong, D., Toleman, M. A., Giske, C. G., Cho, H. S., Sundman, K., Lee, K., & Walsh, T. R. (2009). Characterization of a new metallo-β-lactamase gene, blaNDM-1, and a novel erythromycin esterase gene carried on a unique genetic structure in Klebsiella pneumoniae sequence type 14 from India. *Antimicrobial agents and chemotherapy, 53*(12), 5046-5054.

Zarrilli, R., Casillo, R., Di Popolo, A., Tripodi, M. F., Bagattini, M., Cuccurullo, S., . . . Galdieri, N. (2007). Molecular epidemiology of a clonal outbreak of multidrug-resistant Acinetobacter baumannii in a university hospital in Italy. *Clinical Microbiology and Infection, 13*(5), 481-489.

Zarrilli, R., Crispino, M., Bagattini, M., Barretta, E., Di Popolo, A., Triassi, M., & Villari, P. (2004). Molecular epidemiology of sequential outbreaks of Acinetobacter baumannii in an intensive care unit shows the emergence of carbapenem resistance. *Journal of clinical microbiology, 42*(3), 946-953.

Zarrilli, R., Giannouli, M., Tomasone, F., Triassi, M., & Tsakris, A. (2009). Carbapenem resistance in Acinetobacter baumannii: the molecular epidemic features of an emerging problem in health care facilities. *The Journal of Infection in Developing Countries, 3*(05), 335-341.

Zarrilli, R., Vitale, D., Di Popolo, A., Bagattini, M., Daoud, Z., Khan, A. U., . . . Triassi, M. (2008). A plasmid-borne blaOXA-58 gene confers imipenem resistance to Acinetobacter baumannii isolates from a Lebanese hospital. *Antimicrobial agents and chemotherapy, 52*(11), 4115-4120.

Zhu, L., Yan, Z., Zhang, Z., Zhou, Q., Zhou, J., Wakeland, E. K., . . . Li, Q.-Z. (2013). Complete genome analysis of three Acinetobacter baumannii clinical isolates in China for insight into the diversification of drug resistance elements. *PLoS One, 8*(6), e66584.

Ziha-Zarifi, I., Llanes, C., Köhler, T., Pechere, J.-C., & Plesiat, P. (1999). In Vivo Emergence of Multidrug-Resistant Mutants ofPseudomonas aeruginosa Overexpressing the Active Efflux System MexA-MexB-OprM. *Antimicrobial Agents and Chemotherapy, 43*(2), 287-291.

ABOUT THE AUTHOR

Saba Riaz
Assistant Professor
Department of Microbiology and Molecular Genetics,
University of the Punjab, Lahore, Pakistan
Citi Lab and Research Center, Faisal Town Lahore, Pakistan

Noor Ul Ain
Ph. D Scholar
Department of Microbiology and Molecular Genetics,
University of the Punjab,
Lahore, Pakistan

Dr. Farhan Rasheed
Assistant Professor
Department of Pathology, Allama Iqbal Medical College,
Lahore.

Shahida Hussain
Ph. D Scholar
Department of Microbiology and Molecular Genetics,
University of the Punjab,
Lahore, Pakistan

Hayat Haider
Ph. D Scholar
Department of Microbiology and Molecular Genetics,
University of the Punjab,
Lahore, Pakistan

Samyyia Abrar
Ph. D Scholar
Department of Microbiology and Molecular Genetics,
University of the Punjab,
Lahore, Pakistan